THE BABY MAKERS

Jack Challoner

THE BABY
MAKERS

Jack Challoner

First published 1999 by Channel 4 Books,
an imprint of Macmillan Publishers Ltd
25 Eccleston Place, London SW1W 9NF,
Basingstoke and Oxford

Associated companies throughout the world

ISBN 07522 17011

A CIP catalogue record for this book is available from
the British Library.

Typeset by SX Composing DTP, Rayleigh, Essex
Printed by Mackays of Chatham, PLC

This book accompanies the television series *The Baby Makers* made
by Mentorn Barraclough Carey for Channel 4.
Executive producer: Eamonn Matthews

This book is dedicated to the memory of my father,
Ken Challoner, 1912–1998.

ACKNOWLEDGEMENTS

I would like to acknowledge various people who helped to make this book possible. Thanks to Eamonn Matthews (producer of the television series) and Marian Lacey (production manager) at Mentorn Barraclough Carey; Liz Corrigan at the Centre for Reproductive Medicine, Bristol, UK; and Barney Wyld at the Human Fertilization and Embryology Authority. Thanks also to Jules Acton and Christine King – without their diligence, this book would be incomplete and inconsistent. I would also like to acknowledge the support of my friends and family – in particular Daniel Brookman, Karen Darling and Anne Scully; and my mother, who let me write this book on the dining table when I was 'between houses'.

CONTENTS

INTRODUCTION

Nature has been making babies for the human race unassisted for as long as we've existed. But in the last thirty-odd years, we have learned to understand the complex processes involved in conception and – crucially – to manipulate them. For the first time in our history, we can make fundamental changes to our biological destiny. Not only do we have techniques that can overcome natural infertility, we can also change the very genetic make-up of the babies we are hoping to create.

Most of us have grown used to the idea of IVF — *in vitro* fertilization – where sperm and egg are brought together in a glass dish in the laboratory. But in recent years the technology seems to have exploded in all directions, opening up undreamed-of possibilities. This book grew out of the Channel 4 TV series *The Baby Makers*, a timely look at the amazing developments in this field – and the human stories behind them. The subject is inseparable from the ethical issues that it throws up, challenging as it does long-held assumptions and beliefs about human life. Over the years, it has stimulated countless heated debates between scientists, religious bodies, politicians, journalists – passionate champions of the new technology and equally passionate opponents, and all those who are somewhere in the middle. In this highly sensitive arena, I have aimed to be objective, giving due weight to all shades of opinion. I have drawn on many of the interviews conducted by the TV team with the main players in the field, and used them in conjunction with my own research into the subject.

On the strictly scientific side, it's a complex story, unavoidably involving a fair amount of jargon. For readers whose knowledge of the workings of the human body is what they've half-remembered from school biology lessons, I have outlined the basics in Chapter 1, which also gives a context for the IVF story. That story begins in earnest in Chapter 2, which deals with the incredible medical and scientific work that made IVF possible. Chapters 3–5 follow the gestation of IVF to its triumphant achievement of the first 'test-tube baby' and the aftermath. Chapter 6 concentrates on the ethical and legal issues raised by these unprecedented developments — and Chapter 8 picks up on them later. The other chapters describe the fantastic, almost science-fiction-like variations on the main theme, concluding with a look at cloning and where that may take us in the future.

A note on terminology: I have used the word 'sperm' for the male sex cell, instead of the more proper term 'spermatozoon'. In most cases, I have used the word 'sperms' as the plural of 'sperm'. Where I felt it was appropriate, however, I have used the word 'sperm' as a plural. (This is similar to using the word 'buffalo' as both singular and plural: you normally describe a small number of 'buffaloes', but many 'buffalo'.) As I said, jargon is unavoidable in describing highly complex, sophisticated techniques, but I have tried to make the scientific terms clear. There is a Glossary on page 163 – which also lists the inevitable acronyms used in this field.

Chapter 1

THE FACTS OF LIFE

'The history of a man for the nine months preceding his birth would, probably, be far more interesting and contain events of far greater moment than all the three score and ten years that follow it.'

Samuel Taylor Coleridge

The changing face of reproduction

The business of reproduction is undergoing fundamental change. Before 25 July 1978, all human beings ever born had been conceived in the natural way: by the fertilization of female eggs by male sperms, inside women's bodies. Since that date – which is marked by the birth of the first 'test-tube baby' – ever-increasing numbers have been conceived through fertilization outside the body: *in vitro*, literally 'in glass'. In these cases, the embryo produced after fertilization is transferred to the female patient's womb, where it is hoped that it will develop into a foetus and then a baby. In Britain alone, more than 30,000 babies have been born as the result of IVF.

For couples who are desperate for children of their own but are otherwise unable to have them, successful *in vitro* fertilization (IVF) brings of course profound satisfaction. It is worth bearing in mind, however, that at present the success rate of IVF in infertile couples is about the same as the rate of conception by natural means in the fertile. So, for the many couples for whom IVF does not work, the procedure becomes nothing more than a source of yet more frustration. And it is probably more frustrating still for those who cannot gain access to the treatment – perhaps for financial reasons. The treatment is expensive, and in most cases is paid for by the patients themselves. The availability of state funding for IVF treatment does vary from country to country: in France, for example, women are entitled to at least four state-funded attempts at IVF treatment.

Nevertheless, more and more couples are seeking help to overcome their infertility through IVF treatment. In countries where IVF has been offered for many years, the number of clinics is fairly well matched to the demand, and the increase in supply of the treatment is levelling off. There are other countries, however, where IVF has only relatively recently been introduced, and in which the number of IVF clinics is still growing fairly rapidly. In India, for example, the first IVF baby was born in 1987; ten years later, there were nearly thirty IVF clinics – eight of them in Bombay alone. The popularity of IVF and related techniques is unlikely to decrease in the foreseeable future.

Getting down to basics

So, where do babies come from? No doubt you'll be well acquainted already with enough facts to be going on with, but, to fully appreciate these new technologies, you'll need to know what goes on at a microscopic level. To follow this explanation of human reproduction, you might find it helpful to look at the diagrams of the normal human male and female reproductive systems.

Nature creates a new human life through the union of a sperm and an egg, normally inside a woman's fallopian tubes. The sperms are produced in a very long coiled tube called the epididymis, one of which is found in each testicle. During sexual intercourse, many millions of sperms are released from the epididymis and mixed with a fluid that contains essential nutrients for the sperms. When this mixture of sperms and fluid, semen, is ejaculated into a woman's vagina, sperms are transferred into the female reproductive system. The average volume of semen in each ejaculation is about 4 millilitres, and there are normally about 50 million sperms in each millilitre. Sperms have tails, which they use to propel themselves along, in much the same way as a tadpole uses its tail. The sperms swim in all directions, and some of them travel up through the uterus and into the fallopian tubes.

Meanwhile, the egg has been making a journey of its own. Eggs, or ova, originate from a woman's ovaries. The ovaries are the female sexual organs. They are just less than 3 centimetres across, but they contain hundreds of thousands of potential eggs, called oocytes. Women do not produce new oocytes, as men produce new sperms; instead, they are born with a lifetime's reserve of them. Once each month of a woman's reproductive life, normally one oocyte 'ripens' in response to hormones (explained below). An oocyte begins its ripening process in a fluid-filled sac called a Graafian follicle. It is released from the follicle, and then from the ovary – the process known as ovulation – and makes its way along the fallopian tube towards the uterus. Not until the oocyte is some way along the fallopian tube can it be fertilized. The sperms that find their way up the fallopian tubes blindly swim about and, by chance, a few of them come into contact with the egg. The scene is set for fertilization, and the possible creation of a new human being.

Sperms and eggs are cells, just like the 100 trillion or so other cells that make up an adult human being. Cells are the building blocks of all living things. (Incidentally, the word 'cell' was coined more than 300 years ago, by the Irish microscopist Robert Hooke, who observed that cork seemed to be made from tiny compartments that he likened to monks' cells in monasteries.) Your body is made up of many different types, including skin cells, muscle cells and blood cells. The later illustrations show different types of human cell, allowing us to compare their size and other attributes. An egg cell is surrounded by a layer called the zona pellucida, or zona for short. When a sperm encounters the zona, it is stimulated to release chemicals that allow it to penetrate the zona, entering the space between the zona and the egg itself. Typically, several sperms make it this far, but normally only one goes on to penetrate the egg. This penetration begins when one sperm, still swimming, meets the outer surface of the egg – the cell membrane. Part of the membrane engulfs the sperm, drawing it inside the cell. Almost instantaneously, chemical reactions inside the egg prevent the entry of any more sperms.

An intimate meeting
Once inside the confines of the egg, the sperm begins to disintegrate, releasing genetic material, DNA, from its nucleus. The importance of DNA is explained below – which helps in understanding the techniques described later: pre-implantation genetic diagnosis (Chapter 7), cloning (Chapter 10) and genetic engineering (Chapter 11).

The fertilized egg is called a zygote; a day or so after initial egg—sperm contact, it divides into two identical halves. This process of division is called cleavage, and the cleaved zygote is the embryo. The embryo continues to travel down the fallopian tube towards the uterus. The cells that make up the embryo are still dividing; by the sixth day – when the embryo has grown to the sixteen-cell stage, called a blastocyst – the cells have begun a process called differentiation.

Differentiation is the process by which some of the cells become specialized: until this stage, embryonic cells can develop into any type of cell, such as blood cells or muscle cells. The cells on the outside of the blastocyst go on to form the placenta as they continue to multiply. For a successful pregnancy to occur, these cells must attach themselves to the lining of the uterus (the endometrium), a process called implantation. The rate of differentiation picks up after two weeks, and the cells in the centre of the still-dividing embryo begin to change to specialized cells that will form the various tissues of the developing human being. After eight weeks, the embryo becomes a foetus, which gradually begins to look like a tiny person.

As we shall see, IVF treatment involves intervention in this natural process. In IVF, fertilization takes place outside women's bodies, in glass dishes in a laboratory. Embryos are transferred directly into the womb, with the hope that they will implant and develop normally. In both the natural process and in IVF there is a chance that the embryo will not implant, and will be lost when the woman has her next period. It is thought that embryos that do not implant have certain defects that a woman's body can often somehow detect.

What makes eggs and sperms – the so-called sex cells or 'gametes' – different from other cells? The crucial difference lies in the nucleus of the cell, which contains the genetic material called DNA. Eggs and sperm cells contain only half as much DNA as the other cells of a human body. An embryo has a complete, unique, set of DNA: half from the sperm and half from the egg. So, what is DNA and how does it work?

The importance of DNA

The full name of DNA is deoxyribonucleic acid. This chemical carries the genetic information that makes us human and unique. It makes us who we are. To understand how this can be, it is necessary to consider what DNA is made of. Everything, including DNA, is made of atoms, tiny particles far too small to be seen. Water, for example, is made of two types of atom joined together in groups called molecules. Water molecules are so small that even a tiny drop of water consists of countless millions of them. Each molecule of water is made up of two hydrogen atoms (H) and one oxygen atom (O). (This is why the scientific formula for water is H_2O.) DNA consists of much larger and more complex molecules. Each DNA molecule is made of atoms of the elements carbon, hydrogen, oxygen, nitrogen, phosphorus and sulphur. The illustration on page the central pages of this book shows a typical DNA molecule.

The DNA molecule is long and thin, and it is found in the nucleus of nearly every cell of every living thing. It has the famous 'double helix' structure, resembling a very tall, continuously twisted ladder. Unlike water molecules, which have a fixed constitution (H_2O), DNA molecules differ from each other. The differences lie in the groups of atoms called bases: there are four different types of base that pair up to form the rungs of the ladder. Ultimately, DNA is a long chain of these base pairs. The sequence of bases along the DNA molecule effectively carries all the biological information about the living thing whose cell nucleus it inhabits. Indeed, it is the information in an organism's DNA that makes that organism what it is. The physical characteristics of every living thing are determined by the sequence of bases along the length of its DNA.

Human DNA is, understandably, very complicated: it consists of about 3000 million base pairs. Put poetically rather than scientifically, the DNA bases are like the letters that form the words of the book of a life. DNA has been compared to a recipe book or a build-a-living-thing instruction manual. Our DNA determines the species to which we belong; our hair, eye, and skin colour; our height; our gender; and so on. About 99 per cent of a chimpanzee's DNA is identical to that of a human being, as we are very closely related in evolutionary terms. For two unrelated human beings, the figure is about 99.95 per cent. Two organisms with identical DNA are called clones – so, strictly speaking, identical twins with their same DNA could be called clones. In the future, it is possible that human clones will be produced by genetic engineering. Cloning has already been carried out successfully on other mammals, most notably sheep and cows.

The march of the chromosomes

The entire collection of DNA of a particular organism is called the organism's genotype. It is divided into separate pieces called chromosomes, first observed in 1842. (The name means 'coloured bodies': chromosomes were named in 1888, when coloured dyes were first being used as stains, to help distinguish between different parts of cells under a microscope.) Chromosomes are normally invisible through a low-power microscope, but become visible when a cell is about to divide.

Most cells of a human being contain two sets of twenty-three chromosomes: one set from the mother and one from the father. So, there are a total of forty-six chromosomes in a normal human cell. Sperms and eggs contain only one set of twenty-three chromosomes. When an egg and sperm meet, they create a new genotype, with forty-six chromosomes in total, which can go on to produce a unique human being.

The production of an egg – with twenty-three chromosomes – is called oogenesis. Inside the Graafian follicle, the 'primary oocyte' from which the egg forms contains *two* copies of each of the forty-six chromosomes present in a normal cell. During oogenesis, the oocyte divides twice, eventually forming the mature egg with its twenty-three chromosomes. In the process, two 'polar bodies' are formed, which look like tiny versions of the egg itself. Under a microscope, the two sets of chromosomes can be seen literally being dragged in opposite directions – Robert Edwards, one of the pioneers of IVF technology, described this process as 'the march of the chromosomes'. A similar process (spermatogenesis) results in the production of sperm cells inside a man's epididymis.

The information along the length of DNA molecules, which determines individual characteristics, is expressed in specific regions of DNA called genes. There are thousands of genes in each chromosome, and about 100,000 genes in total in the genotype of a human being. All of the genes concerned with gender are found on the sex chromosomes. There are two types of sex chromosome: X and Y. A fertilized egg containing two X chromosomes will give rise to a female, while an X and a Y will give rise to a male. It is not possible for a fertilized egg to contain two Y chromosomes, since one set of chromosomes has come from the woman, who has two X chromosomes.

Scientific knowledge of human genes is rapidly growing, and some of the implications of this will be described later in the book.

Chemical messengers: hormones

There is one more element of the story of human reproduction that we need to consider before we can confidently explore the technology involved in IVF: the influence of hormones. Hormones play an orchestrating role in reproduction – and in IVF. Some hormones are like chemical switches, turning on or off certain subtle functions of the body by their presence or absence.

One important example is gonadotrophin-releasing hormone (GnRH), also known as luteinizing hormone-releasing hormone (LHRH). This is produced by certain brain cells (neurones) normally in spurts every eighty minutes. As its name suggests, GnRH stimulates the release of certain 'gonadotrophins' – hormones that affect the gonads (ovaries or testes). GnRH causes the release of gonadotrophins called follicle-stimulating hormone (FSH) and luteinizing hormone (LH) from the pituitary gland into the blood stream. In women, FSH causes an oocyte to mature inside a Graafian follicle. As explained earlier, a matured oocyte becomes an egg. Incidentally, men produce FSH, too. It stimulates the production of sperm in the testes. Artificially produced FSH is used in fertility drugs to help some women who do not ovulate and men whose sperm production is low. Large doses of it are often used in IVF, to encourage the ovaries to mature several eggs at the same time. LH causes the Graafian follicle to become a structure called the corpus luteum, described below.

Another important gonadotrophic hormone is human chorionic gonadotrophin (hCG). It is produced by the placenta, which surrounds the foetus and attaches it to the wall of the womb. So this hormone is present only in pregnant women, and its presence is searched for in standard hormone-based pregnancy tests. The placenta forms the bridge between the mother-to-be and the developing foetus. The role of hCG is to maintain the corpus luteum, which fills the empty follicle from which the fertilized egg was released. If there is no hCG, the corpus luteum degenerates. The corpus luteum secretes yet another hormone, called progesterone, that encourages the endometrium (the lining of the uterus) to prepare for implantation. If pregnancy is achieved, the resulting placenta will secrete hCG. The hCG will maintain the corpus luteum, which will produce a constant supply of progesterone. This will maintain the endometrium. In addition, progesterone prevents the production of any more eggs. If the embryo fails to implant, no hCG is produced and the corpus luteum degenerates. With no corpus luteum, no more progesterone is produced, and the endometrium is shed: this is a woman's period.

The interaction of the hormones that make up this cocktail of chemical messengers is vital in human reproduction, and it must be understood, monitored and often altered if IVF is to be successful.

Infertility
The force behind the development of IVF was the drive to overcome infertility: to relieve the pain and frustration of those who want children but whose bodies do not function in the right way. There are

many causes of infertility. Some conditions can be diagnosed directly: a man's epididymis may be blocked by infection, for example, preventing the production of sperm; while one common cause of infertility in women is blocked or severely damaged fallopian tubes. Some women's tubes are blocked from birth, while others become so after pelvic inflammatory disease (PID). The main causes of PID are infectious diseases, notably chlamydia. Another common cause of female infertility is polycystic ovary syndrome (PCO), where a woman produces greater than normal amounts of male hormones (androgens). These hormones, mainly produced by the ovaries themselves, are converted to oestrogen, a female hormone that inhibits ovulation.

In around 30 per cent of infertile couples, however, the cause of infertility is not so easily discernible. In such cases, the World Health Organization defines an infertile couple as a man and woman who do not achieve conception after two years of unprotected intercourse. In practice, though, it is generally accepted that eighteen months of fruitless attempts is enough to indicate infertility (often referred to as 'subfertility'). In many of these cases, poor sperm production or failure to ovulate is discovered to be the reason. Another common cause of infertility in women is endometriosis, the formation of cysts in the lining of the uterus. Couples or individuals may be treated for infertility in a number of different ways, including fertility drugs or surgical procedures. In some cases, they may be referred to a clinic specializing in 'assisted conception', IVF being the best-known technique.

Fertility naturally decreases with increasing age. Women of thirty-five are on average half as fertile as those of thirty-one. Some infertile women in their late thirties are simply experiencing an earlier-than-average menopause, when their reproductive function ceases: eggs no longer mature in their ovaries. Subfertility has also been linked to external factors, such as pollution, alcohol, tobacco and illicit drugs. Stress and anxiety – leading to so-called 'psychosexual dysfunction' – are also potential causes of a failure to produce a child.

The ability to produce offspring is obviously fundamental to the survival of any species, including humans. Many people experience an emotional desire to have children, which is deeper and more complex than a mere drive for sexual intercourse. This desire is so common – across all cultures – that it must be innate. However, nurture also plays a part. Some social and psychological factors may enhance the child-bearing instinct. Among the strongest of these are the expectations of family and friends, the pressure to produce heirs, and the feeling in some that bearing children will bring a sense of purpose to their lives. (Conversely, other social and psychological factors may detract from the desire to procreate – such as career goals, financial status, concern over world population, and sexual orientation.)

Whatever the reasons for the desire to have children, that desire is so strong in many of us that when it cannot be satisfied – when a couple is infertile – it can cause clinical depression, marriage break-ups and even suicide. Here are some anonymous testimonies as to how it feels to be unable to have a much-wanted child:

> 'It binds two people together to have a child between them, and this is what we were looking for, and it wasn't coming.'

> ' "Infertility" is a horrible title. It does something inside you that no one understands unless they have experienced it.'

> 'When you really want a child, and you can't have one, it becomes everything in the world to you.'

> 'You can say, "Oh well, no, I'm never going to feel like that," and then all of a sudden it's the only thing you want in life to have a baby and people that have children very easily perhaps don't understand some of the traumas people go through.'

> 'I think that it's if somebody said to me, "Cut off your right arm and we will guarantee you a healthy baby," I probably would have done that. It's just something that I really, really wanted. I really, really needed it.'

One of the scientists involved in IVF since the early years is Simon Fishel. He set up an organization called the Rachel Foundation, named after the biblical character, explaining:

> 'Rachel said, "Give me a child else I die." Now most people would believe that is simply the cry of the infertile to desire a child, to have a family. I think Rachel is saying a lot more than that. I think Rachel was also saying that life without children is not just worthless but "Without a child I die, genetically, my lineage stops, there is nothing after me."'

The techniques used in IVF

The service provided by IVF centres varies from clinic to clinic. The following overview describes the main elements typically involved in the procedure.

Each attempt at IVF is called a cycle. The initial stage is the suppression of the woman's natural menstrual cycle by controlling the hormonal environment inside her body. This is called down-regulation, and is normally achieved using drugs administered by a nasal spray. These drugs inhibit the production of follicle-stimulating hormone (FSH).

Next, doctors administer drugs that stimulate the ovaries to develop several Graafian follicles, inside which eggs will mature. These drugs normally contain synthetic versions of FSH and luteinizing hormone (LH). When the follicles have reached a certain size, another drug – a synthetic version of the hormone hCG – is injected to ripen the eggs. The eggs are removed from the follicles, using a long syringe called an aspirating needle, which is inserted through the wall of the vagina or, in some cases, through the urethra. The syringe sucks out the fluid that fills the follicles, and the eggs along with it. The positions of the follicles and the needle are monitored throughout this procedure using ultrasound. Between five and twelve eggs are typically retrieved.

The eggs are then transferred to a glass dish where they are mixed with sperms collected, normally, by masturbation. The sperms generally come from the female patient's male partner, although in cases where the woman and man are both infertile they may come from a donor. The sperms are retrieved from the semen by washing it and spinning it in a centrifuge. Only the strongest, most vigorous sperms remain after these processes. Anything up to many thousands of sperms are mixed with each egg in a dish, which is placed in an incubator overnight at a temperature similar to that inside the human body.

The next day, staff at the clinic search for embryos under the microscope. After another day, up to three of any resulting embryos – now consisting of between two and six cells – are transferred to the woman's uterus. There are often serious risks associated with multiple pregnancies, so in most cases only two embryos are transferred. The hope is that one or more will implant, and develop naturally to become a foetus, and eventually a healthy baby.

Any unused embryos may be frozen and used in further attempts if the first cycle is unsuccessful. This avoids the need for further intrusion into the woman's body to retrieve more eggs. In Britain, frozen embryos are retained for up to five years, after which the patients are consulted about what should be done with them. After ten years, they are allowed to thaw, and are disposed of.

Two weeks after the embryos are transferred into the uterus, a standard pregnancy test reveals to the anxious couple whether the IVF cycle has been successful.

There are several variations of the standard IVF technique, some of which will be discussed later in the book. These include:

• Natural cycle IVF
No fertility drugs are given: this is perhaps safer, but results only in the production of the normal one egg per cycle. (See Chapter 3.)

• ICSI (intracytoplasmic sperm injection)
An individual sperm is injected directly into the egg. A recent variation of ICSI, licensed only in some countries, uses immature sperm (spermatids) taken from the male partner's testes. (See Chapter 9.)

• SUZI (sub-zonal insemination)
Several sperms are injected into the region between the zona and the membrane of the egg. (See Chapter 8.)

• IVF using donated gametes (eggs/sperms) or embryos
The name is self-explanatory. This process can used in many different situations: for example, egg-donation if the woman does not produce eggs when her ovaries are stimulated; sperm-donation if the man is infertile; or if there is a risk of one or both partners passing on a serious inherited disease. (See Chapter 7.)

Other 'baby-making' services that some clinics offer – not involving fertilization outside the body – are:

• GIFT (gamete intrafallopian transfer)
Sperms and eggs (gametes), rather than a two-day-old IVF embryo, are transferred into the woman's womb. (See Chapter 8.)

• Donor insemination (DI)
First successfully carried out more than 200 years ago, this technique

involves the transfer of sperm from either the woman's partner or from an anonymous sperm donor into the woman's reproductive tract. The term 'donor insemination' is a collective label for the older terms artificial insemination by donor (AID) and artificial insemination by husband (AIH).

• Surrogacy

In cases where a woman is not physically able to carry a pregnancy to term, another woman – the surrogate mother – carries a child on her behalf. The surrogate may be inseminated with the sperm of the patient's husband; or the couple may have undergone IVF treatment and produced an embryo from their own egg and sperm – in this case the embryo is transferred to the surrogate's womb.

The following three chapters review the momentous developments that made IVF possible.

Chapter 2

A NEW CONCEPTION

'I think all this area, scientific medicine, depends on a fundamental understanding of the basic events in whatever we are studying, whether it is the growth of the follicles, the growth of the embryo, how the embryo attaches to the mother, how it grows in the mother.'

Robert Edwards

The birth, in 1978, of the first human being to be conceived by fertilization outside the body was the culmination of a long scientific struggle – along with a battle for public approval. The team that succeeded in winning through these adversities, and getting IVF to work, was led by biologist Robert Edwards and gynaecologist Patrick Steptoe. The later stages of their work – including the birth of the first 'test-tube baby' – took place in Oldham, in the United Kingdom. These two pioneers were helped enormously in their task by colleagues and friends, and of course by the infertile women who volunteered to take part; also, there were a handful of others attempting IVF in other countries. But the story of the development of IVF really belongs to them. Both Edwards and Steptoe were the subject of frequent opposition from the media and from within the medical and scientific communities, which had to be convinced of the merits of the work they were doing. Edwards in particular felt isolated; he spent much time in hospitals, which removed him, physically and ideologically, from the academic community of which he was part.

The embryonic career

Steptoe did not join Edwards until 1968. Edwards studied agriculture at the University of Bangor in Wales before moving to the field of animal reproduction, which interested him more than his studies of wheat and barley seeds. In 1951, he changed to zoology at Bangor, and was afterwards accepted for postgraduate study at the Institute of Animal Genetics at Edinburgh University. It was at Edinburgh that Edwards laid much of the groundwork of what would become his life's quest. He was more interested in mammals, including humans, than in the fruit flies and simple bacteria that were more commonly used in experiments relating to genetics – the study of inheritance, which involves DNA that makes up chromosomes and genes. Most of the research at the Institute involved mice – mammals that reproduce quickly and in large numbers – and Edwards was inspired by a lecture about experiments on the reproduction of mice. It was given by Alan Beatty, who was the first to transfer fertilized eggs from one mouse to another. Edwards recalls:

> 'So I went to hear a lecture by this young doctor who came in: Dr Beatty... And he was exposing the egg to high temperatures and low temperatures, just at the moment of ovulation: quite brilliant work in view of the knowledge we had at that time, because the knowledge of ovulation and fertilization was so small. And he got these embryos and managed to make chromosomes that were doubled or halved or all sorts of things... it could have been the beginning of a new farming revolution... In the end it didn't work that way, but at the time it was exciting. I thought, "This is it for me," so I said, "Will you take me for a PhD?" He said okay, and we were off: the beginning of my career.'

Edwards's PhD work, based at a research facility called the 'Mouse House', also in Edinburgh, involved affecting the chromosomes of mouse sperm, and investigating the results of fertilization using the altered sperm. Already, ethical questions relating to genetic engineering in eggs and sperms (gametes) became pertinent. However, work on mice and other 'lower animals' was commonplace, and so Edwards was not put under pressure to halt his research – as he would be later on when carrying out experiments involving humans.

At the Mouse House, Edwards fertilized hundreds of mice by artificial insemination. This usually went on into the night, when mice are most active sexually. So Edwards was pleased when he heard of a technique that encouraged female mice to produce ripe eggs at any time. The technique employed an equivalent of the hormone hCG, which stimulates the ripening of eggs in human ovaries. Edwards used the hormone concoction to produce huge numbers of eggs that could be fertilized at any time of the day. The thought crossed his mind that women could be made to produce large numbers of eggs (superovulate) in a similar way, as a method of overcoming some forms of infertility. Nowadays, this is indeed a popular treatment.

The superovulation that Edwards had induced into his mice allowed him to gain access to large numbers of mouse eggs, which enabled him to study ever-increasing numbers of mouse embryos, at any time of the day. He was delighted when one day he and his colleague Alan Gates managed to observe the ripening of an egg under the microscope – exactly two hours after the final injection of the hormone. The two scientists watched excitedly as the chromosomes in the egg cell's nucleus moved about, splitting into two half-sets. Only one of these half-sets of chromosomes remained in the egg, making the egg ready to receive another half-set of chromosomes, from the sperm of a male mouse.

Germ of an idea

Edwards's fascination with the role of chromosomes in reproduction in general – and embryology in particular – was timely: the 1950s had seen rapid progress in the understanding of chromosomes. For example, the molecular structure of DNA – of which chromosomes are composed – was determined in 1953, by Francis Crick and James Watson; and the links between chromosomal abnormalities and congenital medical conditions such as Down syndrome were rapidly being discovered. Edwards was fascinated, and guessed that many of these conditions were related to the way that the chromosomes developed in the ripening egg, but at this stage there was no way that he could carry out research on human eggs: where would he get them from? Despite his fascination with these issues, and with human reproduction in general, Edwards moved in a slightly different direction: into immunology – the study of the immune system. This work took him for a time to California, but on his return to Britain – in a research post at the National Institute for Medical Research in Mill Hill, London – he moved back to embryology, and soon began to think seriously about applying some of what he had learned about mice to humans. He recalls:

'Several reasons we went into humans from mice. I think the most important one was probably the sheer lack of knowledge of the human situation. By the 1950s we were beginning to think much more widely on things like contraception and on genetics and genetic disease in embryos and it was stimulated very much by the discovery that man had forty-six chromosomes. It was always thought that the human race had forty-eight, but it turned out to be forty-six. And, then they started discovering all sorts of men and women who had extra chromosomes or lacking chromosomes and this led to various difficult conditions.'

In 1960, shortly after the birth of his second daughter, Edwards became aware of the sadness and frustration of a couple of his friends who were infertile. At this point, he wondered whether his work in embryology might one day help couples like these:

'We found out that some of our friends were infertile. . . They kept it to themselves until somebody else told us, probably because they wanted children but couldn't have any. And I hadn't really thought too hard about that before then. But I began to think that this was a problem, so I made enquiries and I began to find that it was a fairly common thing – not a rare thing – and that the gift of children is denied to one in ten couples. That is an awful lot, and I knew that if our techniques and if our ideas came to fruition that we'd at least make a try to do something.'

As a first step, Edwards extended his experiments with mouse eggs, this time adding the hCG hormone directly into dishes containing the eggs in a special mixture called a culture. The culture was a mixture of nutrients that the eggs would require, in order to remain alive and ripen. As before, the chromosomes could be seen clearly splitting up as the eggs ripened ready for fertilization. As any good experimenter does, Edwards had set up a 'control': a dish in which no hCG was present. To his complete surprise, he noticed that the eggs in the control dish ripened in exactly the same way as those that had supposedly been stimulated to do so by the hCG. On reviewing the scientific literature, Edwards realized that this revelation was not new. The American biologist Gregory Pincus, who developed the contraceptive pill, had carried out similar experiments more than twenty years before. He had observed the ripening process in both rabbits' and humans' eggs. If Edwards could confirm Pincus's work, then human eggs could be ripened outside the body and would be ready for fertilization. It was at this point that Edwards saw the real potential for *in vitro* fertilization, and the possibility of new hope for infertile couples.

If Edwards was to take any further his ideas for treating infertility by ripening and fertilizing eggs outside the body, he would need to experiment with human eggs. Pincus had worked from eggs taken from pieces of human ovary that had been removed from a woman's body during surgery. Edwards contacted Molly Rose, the consultant gynaecologist at his local hospital, in Edgware. She was more than happy to help, and remembers that day:

> 'Somebody said, "There's somebody to see you," and I said, "Oh yes, I remember he's coming, gown him up." So he was gowned up and came into the theatre, and I opened the abdomen and saw what was wrong, and gave him a piece of ovary and he became very pale and sat down for a moment and then recovered himself and walked out.'

For the next few months, Edwards left dozens of eggs, from both humans and monkeys, in culture dishes, hoping that they would ripen. He left them for increasing periods of time – eventually much longer than the two hours it took for mouse eggs and the eight hours it took for rabbit eggs to ripen. He remembers: 'It was very disappointing when the eggs wouldn't mature *in vitro*, after twelve hours. . . The egg would simply not move and so we decided finally after adding all the hormones and things we could think of. . . that we should now simply let them go longer.'

Eventually, Edwards left an egg for what he thought was a ridiculously long time: twenty-four hours. At last, he saw the beginning of the ripening process. He waited a further four hours before he looked at the last human egg in the batch, and as expected the process had gone further. The signs of maturation in the human egg were unmistakable. Excitedly, Edwards ran into the next laboratory to give the news to his colleague, Mike Ashwood-Smith, who recalls:

> 'Bob comes rushing in and says, "Look, I think I really do have a developing human egg and I think the chromosomes are" – as he put it – "on the march." Well, they don't really march, of course, but it's a good description, I suppose. . . It was quite beautiful and of course, it meant something too: because here, you actually saw an egg developing without having to go through the addition of unusual chemicals. Here it was developing naturally. . . It meant that it was only a question of time before we should be able to fertilize that egg.'

Edwards later discovered that the ripening process takes thirty-six hours, and in IVF treatment today eggs are removed thirty-five hours after the injection into the woman of hCG hormone, which begins the ripening process. Edwards knew at this point that if he could mature eggs outside the body, then there was no reason why he couldn't fertilize them outside the body, too. He knew that attempting this would horrify some people, and he was subject to hostility from many of the doctors to whom he related his idea. Soon, he was also experiencing hostility from within the Institute where he was working: both the head of his department and the Institute's director told Edwards that they thought fertilization *in vitro* was unethical.

Early frustration
A few months later, Edwards's five-year stint at the Institute was at an end, but he was determined to continue his work with human eggs. In 1963, he began work at the Physiological Laboratory in Cambridge. He experimented with the eggs taken from the ovaries of cows, sheep and – when they became available – of women. A year later, once he had come to understand the ripening process better, he decided to attempt fertilization of a human egg. Studies of fertilization *in vitro* using eggs from other species had been carried out by several other scientists, but the prevailing assumption was that fertilization could occur only inside the woman's reproductive system. Despite this, Edwards attempted to fertilize a ripened human egg with his own sperm, in a glass dish. He removed the fluid from his semen, and added the sperms to the ripened eggs. The following morning, he observed that one of the sperms had passed through the zona (the outer coating of the egg): the first stage of fertilization. In that particular case, fertilization went no further, and so there was no positive result.

Some months later, in July 1965, Edwards travelled to Johns Hopkins Hospital in New York. During his six weeks there, he made useful progress in his understanding of human eggs. Despite a variety of different approaches, however, he could not achieve the fertilization he was hoping to see.

The first public knowledge of Edwards's work came in November 1965. He published results of his work so far in the medical journal, *The Lancet*. To his surprise, he noticed a prominent article in a British national newspaper, the *Sunday Times*, describing his work. The article mentioned the dismal vision of the future set out in Aldous Huxley's *Brave New World*, in which human lives were no longer made in the natural way, but were instead manufactured outside the body, in factories. This wouldn't be the last time that the spectre of a soulless mechanized future was raised in relation to Edwards's work.

For several months, Edwards carried out more work on animal eggs in Cambridge, and then experimented with human eggs again during another spell in America. Fertilization of human eggs outside the body evaded him. It seemed that it could only take place inside women's fallopian tubes. Frustrated by his lack of success, he tried a cumbersome technique during his time in America: he tried placing sperms in a little container which was inserted into a woman's vagina, and left there overnight. When the container was removed the next morning, the sperms from inside it were used in an attempted fertilization in a glass dish. Even this intricate procedure brought no success. It was with the same idea in mind – that sperm taken from inside the fallopian tubes might be able to fertilize an egg *in vitro* – that he noticed an article in a medical journal. The article was written by the man who would soon be joining Edwards on his quest for IVF: Patrick Steptoe. Steptoe's article described a surgical technique called laparoscopy, which was to become essential in solving the problems of IVF.

A new way in . . .
Steptoe's article, which appeared in the autumn of 1967, grabbed Edwards's attention as he read. The relatively new technique of laparoscopy involved investigating the interior of a woman's abdomen using a long flexible tube, called a laparoscope. (The word 'laparoscope' comes from the Greek words *laparo*, meaning 'flank', and *skopein*, meaning 'to examine'.) A laparoscope is a type of endoscope, a device that is commonplace in modern hospitals. The best-known endoscopes are those inserted into the body through the mouth, and passed down into the oesophagus and further into the digestive system. Endoscopes allow doctors to examine at close hand parts of the interior of the body that would otherwise be inaccessible without surgery. Most endoscopes are inserted into natural bodily orifices, but laparoscopes are inserted through a small incision made near the navel. General anaesthetic is often required, but the effects on a person's body are far less traumatic than a full surgical investigation would be. Furthermore, certain surgical operations can be performed using a laparoscope, including the removal of such organs as the gall bladder, the appendix and the womb as well as the removal of tumours, cysts and polyps. Steptoe was one of the

pioneers in laparoscopy, and had performed hundreds of investigations. In 1959, when the technique was still in its infancy, he had been experimenting on dead bodies that were awaiting post-mortem examination. He had helped to develop the technology involved in laparoscopy, too. Much of his enthusiasm for the technique was due to his dislike of laparotomies – surgical investigations in which the abdomen is opened up, often for purely diagnostic reasons. In many laparotomies, nothing untoward was found, and so many patients had to endure a major operation for no good reason.

Laparoscopy involves making a small incision, then bloating, or inflating, the abdominal cavity to allow room to manoeuvre. The laparoscope itself is inserted through the incision. Like most endoscopes, a laparoscope consists of two fibre optic bundles – similar to those that carry cable television signals – and other tubes that may, for example, carry water or small surgical tools. The fibre optic bundles consist of flexible, hair-thin glass rods along which light can pass. Because the bundles are flexible, the light can travel round corners. Light passes into the body along one bundle, and illuminates the organ or tissue under examination. Some of the light reflected from the tissues passes back up the other bundle, and is focused using an eyepiece like that on a telescope or binoculars. Modern endoscopes, including laparoscopes, often have video cameras attached, so that the view through the eyepiece can be monitored by several doctors and nurses at the same time. The result is a clear view of the tissue in question; the ovaries, fallopian tubes and other abdominal organs become clearly visible and can be manipulated.

Edwards immediately realized the significance to his own work of what was being explained in Steptoe's article: using a laparoscope, sperms could be removed from inside the fallopian tubes, and should then – according to the wisdom of the day – be able to fertilize a mature egg outside the body. If it were not possible to remove sperms, then at least the fluid from the upper reaches of a woman's reproductive system could be removed, and perhaps this could make fertilization possible, when mixed with egg and sperms outside the body. Attempting these procedures would be a good deal less awkward than Edwards's previous experiment using the capsule inserted into the vagina and left overnight, and which had not worked anyway. As Edwards recalls: 'I went down to the physiology library. I'd always gone down there to read, read, read. The same old door still squeaks. I saw this article by a chap called Steptoe. "It's there! I'll phone him," I thought.'

Edwards did telephone Steptoe, and explained what he was trying to achieve. He was half expecting Steptoe to react in the way that nearly all the other doctors had done: to take no interest in the possibility of IVF, and turn him away. However, Steptoe calmly said, 'Let's have a try.' Despite Edwards's initial excitement about the possibility of success in IVF that laparoscopy opened up, and despite the favourable response that he had received from Steptoe, he did not pursue the matter straightaway. Steptoe was working at the Oldham General Hospital, in Cheshire – a long way from Edwards's own home in Cambridge.

'Well, I looked at the address. It was Oldham, near Manchester. I'd grown up as a schoolboy near Manchester. I knew the distance: a long, long way. And my heart sank at the thought. He had the patients and the laparoscopy, and I had the eggs in Cambridge but with no clinical facilities . . . none at all. I would have to travel to Oldham. . . that was a thought for a father of five . . . It was my field or my home life to some extent. . . it meant days at a time in Oldham.'

Six months later, his interest in laparoscopy still alive, Edwards attended a gynaecological conference at the Royal Society of Medicine in London. One speaker at the conference was talking about the problems of multiple pregnancies caused by fertility drugs. He was discussing how convenient it would be to be able to inspect the ovaries, to see how many eggs were developing. The speaker mentioned the possibility that laparoscopy might be of some use. One of the conference delegates then stood up and denounced laparoscopy as a gimmick. However, another man present at the conference claimed that he had performed hundreds of laparo-scopies, with great success. What's more, he had some very impressive slides with him that supported his claim. This man stood up and spoke eloquently in defence of the technique. He offered his slides to the chairman of the conference and, when they were shown, people were convinced. Laparoscopy was indeed a relevant and successful technique. More importantly to our story, Edwards realized immediately who this man was: it was Patrick Steptoe.

One of Steptoe's colleagues at the time was Muriel Harris. She recalls Steptoe discussing the meeting on his return to Oldham:

'He was at the back of the meeting. The speaker said, "Unfortunately, we have no way of seeing when the follicle ripens." Patrick stood up and said, "Rubbish! I can see the follicle and aspirate the eggs out. I can do this." He was a bit of a bighead. . . he always reported on who said what to who at these meetings. And then he said, "Dr Edwards from Cambridge is coming up." '

Chapter 3

A MEETING OF MINDS

'I think that's what really attracted Bob Edwards to my father: he was just so good at using the laparoscope.'

Andrew Steptoe, son of Patrick Steptoe

Patrick Steptoe was a man of great determination, who for many years as a practising gynaecologist both in London and Oldham, had felt frustrated that there was no effective cure for blocked fallopian tubes that were the cause of infertility in so many women. This goes some way to explaining his resolve when faced with the challenge of making IVF work.

Steptoe was born in Witney, Oxfordshire, in 1913. In his early years, he played the organ at his local cinema, and later he would become a concert pianist. During World War II, he worked as a surgeon in the Royal Navy; in 1941, his ship was torpedoed, and sank. He spent two years in a prisoner-of-war camp in Italy. He died in 1988, but his contributions to the field of IVF live on.

During his collaboration with Patrick Steptoe, Robert Edwards travelled a total of more than a quarter of a million miles on his journey back and forth between Cambridge and Oldham. The work began soon after the conference at which Steptoe had so vociferously defended the technique of laparoscopy. Edwards was introduced to Steptoe – 'You never called me back,' Steptoe said. The two men agreed that they would try to make IVF work in humans. IVF had already been achieved in rabbits, and a reproductive biologist called David Whittingham was working on IVF with mice. He reported his findings on 1968: the only mammal that had been successfully fertilized outside the body was a rabbit; as Whittingham explains:

'Fertilization had taken place in the hamster, but the embryos did not continue to develop. So, being able to get another mammal and demonstrate that you could get normal offspring that were subsequently fertile, was further evidence that these techniques could take place outside the body.'

So the stage was set for the technique to be applied to humans. But there were technical difficulties to be overcome. Perhaps the greatest of these was obtaining sperms from inside the woman's reproductive system. In both rabbit and mouse IVF, the sperms were taken from inside the female animal after copulation. This was because when sperms are inside a female mammal's reproductive system, they undergo a process called capacitation that prepares the sperms for fertilization. The details of the process are still not fully understood, but it is a chemical reaction between the sperms and the mucus found inside the female's reproductive tract. It was therefore assumed that only sperms that had been taken from inside the fallopian tubes – or had at least been mixed with the mucus found there – would fertilize an egg. This is why the prospect of using laparoscopy had had such appeal for Edwards: the possibility that a laparoscope could be used to remove sperms from a woman's body after intercourse.

Ironically, this turned out not to be vital in IVF, since it was soon found that sperms could fertilize eggs irrespective of whether they had been taken from a woman's body or not. In IVF today, the sperms are collected by masturbation, and normally receive no treatment other than washing and separation from the fluid in the semen. However, laparoscopy was to make another, longer-lasting contribution to the development of IVF. Previously, Edwards was only able to experiment with eggs that he had matured from ovarian tissue removed during surgery. Obviously, this is not a convenient source of eggs: a woman referred to an IVF clinic is unlikely to relish the thought of having an ovary removed to overcome infertility. By 1969, Steptoe was removing eggs from living ovaries *in situ*, using the laparoscope. In the modern IVF procedure, even this role of the laparoscope has been superseded: eggs are normally removed from an ovary using a long 'aspirating needle'. The needle is pushed through the wall of the vagina, and into a Graafian follicle inside the ovary. The position of the aspirating needle is monitored using an ultrasound probe. The doctor draws the fluid, along with an egg, out through the needle. So laparoscopy eventually became redundant in the recovery of both eggs and sperm. Perhaps, then, the most important contribution that laparoscopy made to the development of IVF was the fact that it brought Edwards and Steptoe together.

Work in progress

Edwards and Steptoe began their work in April 1968, and it would be more than ten years before the first successful birth of a baby produced by IVF. They began their work in a small makeshift laboratory at Oldham General Hospital. The room they were using had been a storeroom, and was less than ideal for their purpose. Edwards had an assistant in Cambridge, Clare Jackson, who would travel to Oldham with him. Jackson moved from Cambridge soon after those journeys began but her successor, Jean Purdy, was to become an essential part of the team. Edwards pays tribute to her:

> 'Often it was necessary to dash up after a nine o'clock lecture in Cambridge, drive to Oldham, like anything, and get ready for an egg collection at two o'clock, and then I had to come back the next day, to be able to give the second lecture. So I could not be in Oldham all the time. We used to alternate, a technician and myself, and. . . a nurse who turned technician, and in a sense turned back to being a nurse again on IVF, was Jean Purdy who, of all the technicians we took up, proved the most faithful one who stayed to the end. And she was the one who made a contribution equal to that of Steptoe and myself.'

The initial approach at Oldham was to mature eggs outside the body, and fertilize them using sperm taken from the fallopian tubes. Steptoe was obtaining the immature eggs (oocytes) in the same way as Edwards's friend Molly Rose had done when she supplied them to him years before at Edgware General Hospital. He took them from ovarian tissue removed from a woman's body during normal surgical procedures. Edwards was still getting a few eggs from other hospitals, too, but still the number of eggs was frustratingly low. Steptoe collected sperms from women's fallopian tubes, with his laparoscope. After a few months with no success, Edwards decided to try ripening the eggs, and adding sperm, in a new culture fluid devised by one of his colleagues, Barry Bavister. The fluid, dubbed by some as 'Bavister's medium', was developed as part of a programme to make IVF work with hamsters. It was a mixture of several substances, including penicillin and a protein extracted from cow's blood. Edwards took some of Bavister's medium to Oldham, and achieved some limited success: sperms could be seen under the microscope pushing through the outer layer (the zona) of some of the eggs. But, tantalizingly, complete fertilization still evaded them. Sometimes, Edwards would take eggs from the hospital in Oldham to his better-equipped laboratory in Cambridge, to ripen them and attempt fertilization in Bavister's medium there. He carried the eggs in a container strapped to his body for warmth. Bavister would sometimes help out, and recalls:

'Bob had been trying to fertilize human eggs. He popped in one day and said, "I hear your medium's doing well. Can I try it on human eggs?" I don't think the entire work took more than three months. Bob was getting poor quality oocytes from hospitals. . . very poor quality: not stimulated, immature, and we didn't know what to look for. No one had seen a human sperm in an egg. Hamster sperms are huge. . . they look very different. We would take a few precious eggs, incubate the sperm, mix them, and go home for dinner. Then we'd come back to see what happened. One night we climbed over the railing. . . Bob had forgotten his keys. . . Then we would climb six flights of stairs up into our attic laboratory. We would take one precious egg and mount it on a slide, the we would fix it and stain it – which would kill it – and look at it. Bob had a wonderful Zeiss microscope. But we didn't know what to look for.'

Later that year, there was a breakthrough. Edwards's old friend Molly Rose telephoned from London and told Edwards that an ovary was about to become available: would he like to have it? In Cambridge, Edwards obtained twelve eggs by maturing oocytes that he had taken from that ovary. Steptoe was 300 miles away, so Edwards could not gain access to sperms taken from within a woman's reproductive system with a laparoscope. So he and Bavister resorted to adding their own sperms to the matured eggs. Sperms were added to nine of the eggs, all of them in Bavister's medium. Ten hours later, Edwards and Bavister returned to the laboratory, and looked through the microscope to see what, if anything, had happened. Bavister remembers the momentous occasion:

'Bob said, "I've got it." I looked through and there were specks in the egg. But they were in different focal planes . . . just some granulation in the egg. So Bob said "darn" or whatever. An hour later we looked at another egg. He said, "You look this time." And there it was. Unmistakable and clear. . . It was midnight and I was tired. I was twenty-five or so, but Edwards was forty-ish and he was bopping off the walls. He had incredible energy. I remember saying, "This is a picture," and pressing the button.'

Some of the pictures they took that night were published in the scientific journal *Nature* in February 1969. At last, Edwards could see what he had only dreamed of for so long: sperms that had made it into the heart of a human egg. Before this time, in the 1930s and 1940s, a few embryologists had claimed that they had observed fertilization of human eggs outside the body, but none had been proved. It is almost certainly true that Edwards and Bavister were the first people ever to bring about and observe human fertilization *in vitro*.

Edwards's experiment showed that sperms did not have to have been inside a woman's body for fertilization to occur. The breakthrough seems to have relied upon Bavister's medium. The important difference between Bavister's medium and others Edwards had tried was its pH: a measure of acidity or alkalinity. The pH scale of values runs from 1 (strongly acidic) to 14 (strongly alkaline). The pH of concentrated acids like those found in car batteries and in one's stomach is as low as 1.5, while some powerful household cleaners have pHs of around 12 or 13. A solution with a pH of 7 is neither acid nor alkaline: it is said to be neutral. Various parts of the human body are very sensitive to pH. For example, the saliva in your mouth must be slightly acidic for chemicals called enzymes to break down nutrients in your food, while blood's pH is automatically stabilized at values of between 7.35 and 7.45. Bavister's medium was more alkaline than other culture fluids that Edwards had tried.

There was a period of nearly a year between that first proper fertilization and the publication of the article in *Nature*. During this time, several other eggs were successfully fertilized *in vitro*, mostly in Oldham. Edwards and Steptoe collected data on their experiments, along with many photographs to back up their claims. At the head of the article, Edwards included a wonderful understatement: 'This may have some clinical uses.'

Inevitable opposition

The team knew that the sort of experiments they were carrying out were accompanied by difficult ethical issues. Not everyone would agree with what they were doing, but they hoped that keeping their discovery within the scientific community would reduce the inevitable pressure from some public commentators to stop them experimenting with the fundamentals of human life. Their hope for anonymity was not realized, however. Immediately after the *Nature* article was published, Edwards's and Steptoe's achievement made headlines in the national and international press and was heavily featured on television. 'Life is created in test tube' read one headline. The phrase 'test-tube baby' became part of everyday language, and IVF was big news. The telephone seemed never to stop ringing, sometimes with congratulations, at other times with endless questions. Barry Bavister recalls the buzz of interest at Cambridge:

> 'When the *Nature* paper was published, TV crews turned up and there were inch-thick cables running up the lab. They had to use outside broadcast units in those days. And journalists rang up other people in the lab at midnight to get reactions. Crews from Germany and Japan were trudging up the five flights of stairs to [Edwards's] office.'

As expected, there were those who publicly voiced their disapproval. The prominent Cambridge zoologist Lord Victor Rothschild clamed that no fertilization had taken place – that the photographs showed something else. Edwards's PhD student at the time, Richard Gardner, remembers what happened:

'There was great hilarity at the time because Lord Rothschild, who had worked for many years on fertilization in the sea urchin, wrote a very pompous letter from the House of Lords saying that. . . the presence of [two nuclei] and a sperm tail was not fertilization, you had to show that the eggs cleaved normally and went well beyond that. . . I had gone to purchase a copy of Lord Rothschild's book and although it was all about fertilization in sea urchin, lo and behold the frontispiece showed a mouse egg with [two nuclei] and a sperm tail, and the caption was: "A living fertilized mouse egg". So I remember Bob and co. wrote a report to Rothschild that was published later which sort of ended up saying, "He's hoist with his own petard: see the frontispiece to his book". I think with the knowledge of hindsight it was probably a slightly foolish thing because Lord Rothschild became pretty vigorously anti this area of reproductive biology subsequently, but it was very entertaining at the time.'

Some of the other critics were members of the religious community, who objected to the experiments on moral grounds. Their objections often centred on the fact that in IVF the reproductive process was removed from the sexual act, and was therefore against the will of God. The ethical and moral debates are considered more closely in Chapter 5. Another fear expressed by some people was that babies born through IVF might turn out to be monsters. This was a very real concern, and it had some scientific weight behind it: what if extra chromosomes found their way into an embryo while it was being manipulated in the laboratory? Edwards exhaustively tested the chromosomes of the eggs that he and Purdy fertilized. He satisfied himself that the rate of chromosomal abnormality was the same as in natural embryos, and this convinced him to carry on. He also knew that a woman's body naturally rejects most embryos with chromosome defects, and he was confident that there would be no difference with embryos created *in vitro*.

After the initial blaze of publicity surrounding the first fertilization, Robert Edwards, Patrick Steptoe and Jean Purdy moved on to the next stage of their work. They had two main practical challenges to overcome. Firstly, they had to find a way to encourage their fertilized eggs to divide. If an egg fertilized outside the body can proceed no further than fertilization, then it can never grow to become a foetus, and so never produce a baby. Secondly, they were determined to use eggs that had matured inside women's bodies. This second point was important because experiments in animal IVF had shown that the development of embryos was impeded when the eggs involved had been ripened outside the body. Furthermore, as already mentioned, it would be more than mere inconvenience for a woman undergoing treatment for infertility to have her ovaries removed for the retrieval of immature eggs. So Patrick Steptoe would remove eggs directly from the Graafian follicles inside the patients' ovaries, using his laparoscope. This would mean involving patients who were willing to volunteer to have eggs removed. Such volunteers were found, and the work continued.

The team established the routine for carrying out their new procedure: hormones were given to patients, to stimulate the ripening of the eggs; then Steptoe removed eggs thirty-six hours later with his laparoscope. John Webster, one of Steptoe's assistants, recalls:

'The eggs were collected laparoscopically in those days, and each of the follicles – the tiny cysts which contained the eggs – was aspirated and the fluid was sent round to Bob and Jean, who sat in a little room next door to the operating theatre. If the egg was identified, Bob or Jean would shout through, "Got the egg, Patrick," and we'd carry on with another follicle.'

After egg collection Edwards added sperms to attempt fertilization of the eggs in a dish containing Bavister's medium. Because Edwards and Bavister had been successful in fertilizing eggs with their own sperms, the team decided to abandon the idea of taking sperms from inside the women's fallopian tubes. Instead, they used sperms produced by the female patients' husbands, by masturbation. Muriel Harris, another of Steptoe's assistants, remembers when 'The husband would come to the theatre. The nurse would give them a pot to fill and show them to the toilet.'

The team managed to fertilize a large number of eggs, and observed how they cleaved and grew. Some of the eggs that the team managed to fertilize developed to the eight-cell stage. In modern IVF treatment, embryos are normally transferred into patients' wombs at this stage, but it was important for the team to observe at least the next stage of embryo development. Only then could they be certain that embryos produced outside the body had a chance of developing once transferred. However, no such development was observed. The team even tried to implant the fertilized human eggs (zygotes) into rabbits' wombs, to give them a better chance of survival. On removal from the rabbits' wombs, the eggs still showed no development beyond eight cells. Eventually, they decided to change the culture fluid, to bring it more in line with conditions inside women's reproductive systems. They found such a fluid, which enabled the fertilized eggs to continue their development, and soon they produced their first blastocysts: embryos at or just beyond the sixteen-cell stage that look like translucent, fluid-filled raspberries. Edwards recalls the achievement:

> 'I remember we were letting the embryos grow from the cleaving stages from forty-eight hours and so on, and after four days in culture, I got a telephone call from Jean who was on duty saying she couldn't understand what's happened to these embryos, they're doing strange things before her eyes. They seemed to be having fluid accumulating in them, making little balls and expanding and things. So I had to fly up, I think it was through the snow, about 200 miles, late at night, into the theatre, and there's the four most beautiful blastocysts, light circular spheres floating, glistening by the light underneath: five days, five and a half days old.'

At the blastocyst stage, an embryo's outer surface is ready for implantation in the lining of the womb. However, although these tiny parcels of life – still smaller than a pinhead – were more than developed enough to be implanted back into the woman from whom the eggs had been taken, the laboratory conditions in which the team was working (now in an old laundry room next to an operating theatre at Oldham General Hospital) were not sterile enough. Besides, there were chromosome tests that had to be carried out – tests that would mean the blastocysts would have to be destroyed. Edwards continues:

'Indeed we'd have transferred those that very night, perhaps we should have done, but we didn't. Because we had to look at them and check a few chromosomes, do the minimum tests that we needed to make sure that things were normal. But it was fantastic, it was absolutely astonishing. And we prepared them for [chromosome tests] at the end of the day, which is desperately sad to have to do that.'

Edwards and Steptoe needed to find a new space that was more conducive to carrying out their work successfully. They made an application for funding to the Medical Research Council (MRC) but, as explained in the response they received, 'the Council came to the conclusion that they could not agree to [the] request for long-term support since they had serious doubts about ethical aspects of the proposed investigations in humans'. Some of these doubts centred on the experimentation with fertilized human eggs, and in particular the transfer of fertilized eggs into women's wombs. They were concerned that it was too soon to attempt this, until studies in other primates, such as monkeys, had been carried out and shown the technique to be safe. Monkeys are genetically similar to humans, and the MRC assumed that their reproductive systems are also similar. However, Robert Edwards knew that this was not true: for example, hormone treatments that were successful in humans and mice did not work in monkeys. The MRC also had reservations about the use of laparoscopy in the IVF experiments. Perhaps some of the Council's advisers were also worried about the moral questions raised by the ultimate death of the embryos that were the subject of research. Many other people – particularly those representing pro-life, anti-abortion groups – expressed their horror about the destruction of embryos, which they saw as potential human beings. To be examined for any chromosomal abnormalities, the embryos resulting from Edwards's and Steptoe's early IVF studies had to be squashed on to a microscope slide, and destroyed. Did Edwards feel that he was destroying human beings, or at least potential human beings? His response:

'They've formed nothing, they're about to start the first step on their life. Now you have to put the value of that against the desperate tribulations of infertility. I never deny it is a life, but it depends what you mean by life. And at this tiny unorganized stage I think that those embryos are far more expendable than later embryos, and if we can use them for research, we have to use them for research.'

There are some important things to take into account when considering the question of whether destroying an embryo is destroying a human being – the equivalent of murder. The moral and ethical questions surrounding the status of an embryo will be looked at later. For now, it is worth mentioning two facts. Firstly, an embryo cannot be considered as a human individual: sometimes an embryo at this stage quite naturally splits, and can form two or more separate, but genetically identical, embryos that both implant. This is how identical twins, triplets and quadruplets are formed. Secondly, and perhaps more importantly, there is no way that an embryo at an early stage can have any feelings: its cells are yet to begin the process of differentiation (see page 3), so the embryo has no nerve cells and certainly no brain. It is also worth noting that a woman's body naturally rejects most embryos that reach this stage. The intra-uterine contraceptive device (IUCD) – a popular method of contraception – is designed to prevent the implantation of embryos, and encourage this rejection. As we shall see in Chapter 6, scientific research involving human embryos is generally permitted up to fourteen days after fertilization.

In 1970, a BBC television programme stimulated more public interest and outcry. Some of the patients at Oldham were hounded by members of the press that were hungry for unique or sensational insight into what was going on. Work was halted for a few months and, by the time it started up again, the team had moved to a better-equipped location. Although the Medical Research Council had refused to fund the work, the Oldham Area Health Authority agreed to lend their support: both financially and by allowing the team to use some rooms in a small hospital. It was called Kershaw's Cottage Hospital and, with the help of local charities and his own money, Steptoe set out to equip it. Edwards was also receiving some financial assistance from the Ford Foundation in America, which had been interested in his work for some time.

Moving on

Muriel Harris remembers that initially, conditions at Kershaw's Hospital were less than ideal:

'It had a disused operating theatre with a small anaesthetic room attached to it. It had been disused for a long time and when I went up to look at it, it was an absolute shambles: it was just full of old junk. It had been used as a storage area really. But . . . I thought we could do something with it. So we cleaned it all out, and made it as aseptic as we possibly could. It was an old place. And next to it, there was a small room which Bob could use as a laboratory. And that was in close proximity to the operating theatre.

'I sort of probed around and found out that Bolton General were refurbishing their theatres, and they were getting rid of their old operating table. So I went to look at it and it was just exactly what I wanted. It was a bit battered about, but I thought we could do something with it. They wanted £50 for it, and eventually when I told them it was for research, and we hadn't got much money, we got it for £25. Providing we transported it away.'

The work at Kershaw's began in 1971. Just as the team was getting ready for their first embryo transfer, Edwards was persuaded to attend a symposium in Washington DC. At dinner the night before the meeting – and, more publicly, at the meeting itself – some prominent experts denounced what Edwards was trying to do. One of these was the celebrated molecular biologist James Watson, who had won a Nobel Prize for his role in the discovery of the structure of DNA molecules. Watson was a member of the panel presiding over the meeting. He told Edwards that he would have to accept the 'necessity of infanticide' if he was to continue his work. He continued: 'What are you going to do with the mistakes?' – an emotionally charged phrase that was to be printed in several newspapers. The point was that until a baby was produced by IVF, one just couldn't know what might happen. Another member of the panel believed that Edwards's work was unethical because of the necessary experimentation with potential human beings. A British embryologist, Anne McLaren, was also on the panel: she was in favour of IVF, but was not convinced that Edwards and Steptoe were ready. (She was later part of the British Committee on Human Fertilization and Embryology – the Warnock Committee – which is discussed in Chapter 6.)

Not everyone present at the Washington symposium was hostile. A friend of Edwards, Howard Jones, who together with his wife Georgeanna would later set up the first IVF centre in the United States, spoke in defence of Edwards's work. Edwards received some enthusiastic support from the audience present at the meeting, too, when he eloquently and unequivocally answered the criticisms that had been levelled at him. 'Well, I told the Presbyterian minister that he was a hundred years out of date and to my astonishment the audience stood and applauded that remark.' Edwards went on from Washington to Tokyo, to another symposium. Australian IVF pioneer Ian Johnston was there. He had just begun to take an interest in IVF, and he came away inspired:

'I went to an international infertility conference in Tokyo in 1971 and Bob Edwards was there showing his fantastic material on the early work that he and Patrick Steptoe were doing with human eggs – collected by laparoscopy – and the sort of work they were trying to do to create embryos and so on and it blew the audience away and me with it, and I thought this is easy. . . this is the technology. We've got laparoscopy, all I need is an embryologist to sort out the laboratory problems and we'll have IVF up and running by 1972.'

Indeed, Ian Johnston set up an experimental IVF programme with Carl Wood, in Melbourne, that was to become world-renowned, and was in competition with the team at Kershaw's to produce the first IVF child. (More of the Australian IVF efforts in Chapter 5.) Edwards returned to England more determined than ever. On his journeys between Cambridge and Oldham, he was still accompanied by Jean Purdy, who has since died. One of the patients at Kershaw's remembers her fondly:

'Jean Purdy was an amazing girl. She was a very kind, considerate, dedicated lady. She had travelled up and down to Oldham with Bob Edwards, I think for years, doing the research work originally and then, to complete the system where the eggs were withdrawn and fertilized in the petri dishes. And it was always Jean that we used to turn to when she was looking after the little dishes. So it was always Jean we would go to and say, "How are they coming along?" She would either give you the thumbs up or she would say, "Well, we've got a little bit longer to wait," but she was kindness itself, she was an absolutely amazing person.'

In December 1971, Patrick Steptoe made the first ever transfer of a human embryo produced by IVF. No longer were the volunteers only having eggs removed: successfully fertilized eggs would be placed inside their wombs if they reached the eight-cell stage of development. Steptoe transferred the embryo using a catheter (a flexible tube) pushed through the cervix and into the womb. The first attempt did not result in a pregnancy: the embryo failed to implant. The rate of fertilization began to drop lower than before and, for a few months, little progress was made. Furthermore, not one embryo would implant. The team supposed that these problems were something to do with hormones. They tried various different combinations of hormone treatments, to control each woman's menstrual cycle and prevent the loss of the transferred embryo. It was important to work out which hormones to inject and when. Getting this right required a good deal of experimentation, and it would not be until the summer of 1975 that they achieved the first pregnancy.

Meanwhile in New York

In the meantime, there were other developments in the world of IVF outside Oldham and Cambridge. Perhaps most significant was the case of Doris del Zio in New York. In 1973, Mrs del Zio could have become the first woman to give birth with the aid of IVF. She and her husband had read that Dr Landrum Shettles, at the Columbia Presbyterian Hospital, had successfully fertilized a human egg outside the body. The couple approached Dr Shettles, in the hope that he could help to give them a child, and he agreed to take up their case. In September 1973, an egg was removed from one of Mrs del Zio's ovaries, and mixed with some of her husband's sperms in a flask in Shettles' laboratory. When the Chief of Obstetrics at the hospital found out what had happened, he was very concerned, on two main counts. Firstly, the experiment had not been approved by the hospital's Human Experimentation Review Board, and secondly – on a more personal level – he believed that there was a high risk that the baby would be a 'monster'. The belief that IVF would result in babies that were monstrously malformed was held by many people at the time – even doctors and scientists. This point of view – now shown to be false – was given credence by the highly publicized comments of James Watson and others at the 1971 Washington symposium, along with various articles that appeared in respected publications such as the *Journal of the American Medical Association*, and the outcomes of various ethical studies. This is not to mention the perception of the media and public at large, that tended to see Edwards and other IVF scientists as equivalent to Dr Frankenstein. So, the Chief of Obstetrics at the Columbia Presbyterian Hospital, driven by these beliefs, took it upon himself to destroy the del Zios' chance of success in the IVF programme. He opened the flask containing the mixture of egg and sperms, which destroyed the culture inside, and, along with it, any chance of the del Zios having a child from this experiment.

The del Zios were horrified. Doris del Zio remembers how she felt:

> 'As far as I was concerned at that time he had murdered my baby, he had taken away any chance of that child developing. . . As far as I was concerned that was my child. I know scientifically maybe it wasn't, but to me it was. He didn't give it a chance, he didn't give it a chance and he didn't give me a chance to be a mother.'

The del Zios sued the hospital, the university of which it is part, and the Chief of Obstetrics, for $1.5 million. After more than five years, the del Zios were awarded $50,000.

Back in Britain, during the years between 1972 and 1974, Edwards concentrated less on the project. For some periods, work halted altogether. Wounded by the criticism and disillusioned by the failure of the team's experiments, he began to concentrate more on politics. He was a city councillor and also stood for election as a Labour Party candidate. He was not elected, and he soon returned to his work at Kershaw's.

Chapter 4

A CHILD IS BORN

'Yes, I feel proud that I was part of it... but I didn't actually help it happen. In a way I'm proud that what I was has helped other people have children.'

Louise Brown

Louise Joy Brown was the first baby to be born as a result of IVF treatment, but her mother, Lesley, was not the first woman to become pregnant by the implantation of an embryo conceived by IVF.

False starts

The first IVF pregnancy was confirmed – by a test for the hormone hCG in the patient's urine – in the summer of 1975. At last, the team in Oldham and Cambridge felt that success was in their grasp. But they and their volunteer patients were to suffer several disappointments over the next three years, before eventual success, culminating in the birth of Louise Brown in 1978. Their first disappointment came just weeks after that first pregnancy was confirmed. When the embryo was about six weeks old, Patrick Steptoe suspected that this was an ectopic pregnancy: one in which the embryo implants in the fallopian tubes instead of inside the womb itself. This sort of pregnancy carries great risks to both patient and embryo: it is likely that the embryo will burst through the fallopian tube as it grows. Despite the fact that the patient had lost most of each of her fallopian tubes through disease and during surgery, the embryo had implanted at the position where the remains of one of the fallopian tubes joined on to the top of the womb. There was a slight swelling at one side of the womb. Steptoe investigated, using his laparoscope, and when he was certain that this was an ectopic pregnancy, he removed the embryo there and then.

The team reported the news of the first pregnancy to the medical journal *The Lancet*, and the work at Oldham once again became the subject of both interest and scorn. Some claimed that the pregnancy had been the result of sperms fertilizing an egg that had somehow managed to make its way down the fallopian tubes: Steptoe and Edwards knew this was not possible, as the tube was not complete. During this time, a BBC television *Horizon* programme examined the progress in, and the prospects for, IVF technology. Robert Winston, a fertility expert, appeared on the programme. Like many in the medical establishment, Winston denounced IVF, suggesting instead that transplants of fallopian tubes offered the best way forward. Winston now admits that he was wrong:

'I genuinely didn't feel at the time what Patrick [Steptoe] and Bob Edwards were doing was really likely to be of great human benefit. I could see its importance scientifically and I went to the lectures thinking that's really very interesting, we'll learn about embryonic development, but I didn't see how this could be actually turned into a successful clinical treatment, and I didn't start to really feel that it might be until about 1980.'

The *Horizon* programme did little to bolster public confidence in IVF. The ectopic pregnancy, too, was a blow for Edwards and Steptoe, although it had shown that they were doing something right. It must have been desperately sad for the patient as well, of course. She had already endured a variety of unsuccessful fertility treatments since 1967 and now, in 1975, she had to suffer the disappointment of having her developing embryo removed and destroyed. She says, 'You know, I wonder sometimes what it was. The way I always have it in my mind was that it was a boy – don't know why.'

Sometimes, ectopic pregnancies occur after normal fertilization inside the body. Nevertheless, the team wondered whether this one had anything to with their procedures: perhaps all embryos transferred after IVF would implant in the fallopian tubes? The second pregnancy answered that question – no: in this case, the patient's fallopian tubes had been removed completely. However, for some reason, the embryo was rejected by the woman's body early in the pregnancy. Again, failure of an embryo to implant is common in those produced naturally, and so this negative result did not necessarily indicate that the IVF procedure was to blame. It was still a disappointment, however, and until the team could achieve a normal, sustained pregnancy – until they achieved a positive result with IVF – they would not know for sure whether their technique could ever work, even in principle.

In from the cold

Shortly after this second pregnancy, while Steptoe underwent a hip replacement operation and the subsequent recovery, Edwards and Jean Purdy discussed various options open to them. These included freezing embryos so that they could be stored until the optimum time for transfer to the womb. A former colleague of Edwards, David Whittingham, had the facilities to freeze embryos, but he was in London, as he recalls:

> 'Bob was in Oldham with the embryos, and I was down in London. So we had to find some means of transporting them. . . and we chose the guard on the train. I would meet [the guard] at Euston Station, obtain the material and take it back to the lab. . . We tried cooling them, and freezing them, and our initial success showed that this was a feasible thing that could be done with human embryos in the future. But the material that we had at the time was limited and this was only an initial look to see whether this could be done when they had all the techniques working to get live babies.'

Freezing – or cryopreservation – of embryos is now routine procedure at IVF clinics. The rationale behind its use in such clinics is that more embryos are produced than are needed, and 'spare' ones are retained and transferred later if the first attempt at IVF fails. Edwards and Purdy had used cryopreservation so that they could choose the best time to transfer the embryos to the patients' bodies. They had no success with the technique, even after obtaining a cryogenics machine to use at Kershaw's.

Another option that the team considered was reducing or eradicating the hCG hormone, administered to patients to stimulate the ripening of oocytes. Normally only one egg matures each month in one of a woman's ovaries, but the number can be increased using certain hormones, including hCG. However, the hCG affected the patients' menstrual cycles in an undesirable way, as John Webster – Steptoe's assistant – remembers: 'The drugs which we were giving to stimulate the ovaries were shortening the menstrual cycle and we felt because of this the embryos weren't getting sufficient chance to implant.'

Using smaller amounts of hormone would perhaps interfere less with the natural menstrual cycle, and might give a better chance of implantation. However, without the hCG, only one egg is produced per cycle. The chance of achieving fertilization with a single egg is obviously less than with several. It would be down to the expertise of Steptoe to recover a single egg; and the expertise of Edwards and Purdy to fertilize that egg. As we shall see, the use of hormones in IVF to control the woman's menstrual cycle, and to stimulate superovulation, was perfected by Carl Wood and Alan Trounson in Australia in the late 1970s, and is now common practice. Nevertheless, Edwards and Purdy decided to try to get closer to 'nature's way', reducing the hCG given to patients. This approach continued for the rest of the experimental programme.

If the team was to rely on ovulation at a time determined by the body's natural cycle – so-called natural cycle IVF – it would be crucial to know exactly when to collect the ripening eggs from the ovaries. What Edwards and Purdy needed was a test for one of the hormones that stimulate the ripening process: leuteinizing hormone (LH). The release of LH – from the pituitary gland – leads to a dramatic increase in the concentration of that hormone present in a woman's urine, the so-called 'LH surge'. If Edwards could test a patient's urine and detect the LH surge, he would be able to work out when the egg would be just mature enough to be removed from the ovary, ready for fertilization. A gynaecologist friend of Edwards in London told him that such a test did exist. It was called Hi-Gonavis, and Edwards used it in conjunction with a more established test, for another hormone, oestrogen, to predict successfully just the right moment to collect the egg. This often meant that the staff at Kershaw's worked odd hours, as one of the nurses describes:

'Steptoe and Edwards had just started getting things sorted at Kershaw's. . . They had to collect the eggs: this could be any time between 9pm and 2am. Steptoe had already explained the procedure to the women when we arrived. It was all very rushed because there was only a very small window to retrieve the egg: you had to enter the follicle at just the right time. We could only work when Bob was on holiday from the university, so when everyone else was on holiday – summer, Christmas and Easter – we worked all day and night: you had to be on call twenty-four hours a day. We were all working between 90 and 120 hours a week. I didn't mind, though, because the work was so interesting, and the team was a very close-knit community.'

Enter the Browns . . .
In November 1977, a number of women were selected for treatment. Most had damaged fallopian tubes, but ovulated normally. An egg was collected from the first woman, fertilized, and the resulting embryo was transferred to the woman's womb once it reached the eight-cell stage. Sadly, the woman menstruated a few days later: the embryo had not implanted. Patrick Steptoe was not able to collect an egg from the third woman, so there was no fertilization, let alone implantation, in her case.

The second woman in the series was Lesley Brown, a twenty-nine-year-old from Bristol. She had been referred to Steptoe by her doctor, Ruth Hinton. Dr Hinton had met Steptoe at a conference in Bristol, and was aware of what he was trying to do. The cause of Lesley Brown's infertility was blocked fallopian tubes: the blockage prevented eggs released from the ovary from meeting any sperms. This was exactly the sort of problem that Edwards and Steptoe hoped that IVF might overcome. An operation in 1970 had failed to reopen Mrs Brown's fallopian tubes. Dr Hinton initially referred Mrs Brown to Steptoe, hoping that he might be able to use laparoscopy to succeed where the previous operation had failed. The Browns travelled to Manchester to meet Steptoe. John Brown's first impression:

'There was a young girl at the desk there and I said, "Mr and Mrs Brown to see Mr Steptoe." "Oh yes, take a seat, sir, he'll see you in a minute." So we sat there. We'd been there about ten, fifteen minutes and this gentleman comes out in a grey suit and there's a booming voice: "Mr and Mrs Brown!"'

During this first consultation, Steptoe asked the couple whether they would like to be involved in the IVF trials that he, Edwards and Purdy were carrying out. The Browns said that they would – they desperately wanted to have a child. Couples taking part in the programme were asked to consent to the abortion of a baby that was not developing safely, or was malformed. So, there was a chance that, if and when a woman on the programme became pregnant, she would have to have her long-awaited pregnancy terminated. The Browns agreed, and in August Mrs Brown underwent the laparoscopic surgery she had been promised; and in November, she and her husband travelled to Oldham again – this time for the beginning of an IVF cycle. The Hi-Gonavis test informed the team of the best time to collect an egg from a Graafian follicle in one of Mrs Brown's ovaries. Just after eleven o'clock on the morning of 10 November 1977, an egg was removed from Mrs Brown's left ovary. At the same time, husband John produced a sperm sample:

> 'Nurse Buckley came in and said, "Hello, John, you can do your little bit now." I said, "Do I have to?" She said, "Well, nobody else can do it. But I can always give you a hand!" I thought, "No thank you!"'

The sperm sample was washed and prepared for mixing with the egg. Back in the operating theatre, Steptoe removed the fluid from the follicle, and a nurse gave it to Edwards in the laboratory next door. Edwards mixed with it some of Mr Brown's sperms. Later that day, the egg was fertilized and, by the following evening, the fertilized egg had cleaved, making two cells where there had been one. By seven o'clock the next evening the embryo was a clump of six cells. The cleaving process continued, and eventually, after midnight, the embryo consisted of eight cells: it was ready for transfer into Mrs Brown's womb.

Steptoe and Edwards transferred the embryo from a syringe, through a long tube called a cannula, into Lesley Brown's womb. Edwards and Purdy examined the syringe and the cannula to make sure that the embryo had been transferred. Over the next few weeks, Mrs Brown gave frequent urine samples, and these were sent to Edwards and Purdy in Cambridge. Tests for hormone levels in the urine seemed to show that Lesley Brown was pregnant, and after about three weeks, Edwards was convinced. He wrote a short letter to Mrs Brown, informing her that the tests showed that she was indeed pregnant. It read: 'Dear Mrs Brown, just a short note to let you know that the early results on your blood and urine samples are very encouraging and indicate that you might be in early pregnancy, so please take things quietly – no skiing, climbing or anything too strenuous, including Xmas shopping. Best wishes, yours sincerely, Dr Edwards.'

Everything continued to indicate that the pregnancy was normal, and the team was excited. They knew that they had to keep the news of the pregnancy secret for now: partly to respect Mrs Brown's privacy, and partly in case something went wrong – the news would have given critics fuel for their objections to IVF. So the pregnancy remained a secret until Mrs Brown's frequent visits would make it obvious. Muriel Harris remembers how she found out the good news:

'One day Patrick Steptoe came into my office and closed the door. "I haven't told anyone else this, but Mrs Brown has had a positive test." Then he said, "Don't tell anyone else." I badgered him to tell the nurses. He agreed – but said, "Keep it close."'

Embryos were transferred into several other patients, but with only one success, in January 1978. After reading a scientific paper concerning the daily cycles of hormone levels, Edwards realized that the time of day might affect whether a transferred embryo would implant. The fact that Lesley Brown's embryo had been transferred in the middle of the night had turned out to be crucial. Most of the other transfers had been carried out during the day. So in an attempt to work around the patients' natural rhythms, as well as to avoid the noisy environment during the busy days, Steptoe usually carried out the embryo transfers late at night. Nowadays, IVF doctors have control over the hormone levels in a patient's body, and so time of day is no longer important for embryo transfer. However, Edwards's idea of transferring embryos at night had brought some success, and in May the team achieved another positive implantation.

Meanwhile, there were a few signs of potential problems with Mrs Brown's pregnancy. The embryo had become a foetus, but was growing slowly; Mrs Brown's blood pressure was high, and worst of all there were signs of toxaemia of pregnancy: a fairly rare condition that causes headaches, visual disturbances and potentially dangerous high blood pressure. However, ultrasound scans showed that the foetus had a beating heart, and seemed otherwise normal. One of the nurses recalls a particular day, when Steptoe used a device called a sonicade to listen for the heartbeat of the foetus inside Lesley Brown's womb.:

'The sonicade was brought and it went into the side ward. And there were three or four in the side ward, but you could hear a pin drop, you could hear the breathing. You could hear the rushing of the blood, you could hear Lesley's heartbeat, which obviously is strong and slow, and then you could hear a very quick rapid heartbeat. And Mr Steptoe came out of the side ward and he never said a word. He had this pleasant smirk on his face, and he just walked off the ward, which was so unusual for him: he usually went back in the office for coffee and discussion on what to do next and he just walked off the ward. And the senior registrar said to Sister in the corridor, "I think history has been made today." And I don't think we realized just what we'd witnessed.

You know, even though we knew Lesley was pregnant, to actually be there was just something else.'

An amniocentesis test carried out on fluids taken from around the foetus ruled out so-called neural tube defects, such as spina bifida. A different test carried out on the same fluid examined the chromosomes from the growing foetus. The results of this test arrived while Steptoe was away on holiday, on board a cruise ship. So the hospital secretary, Diana Mann, sent a radio-telegram to the cruise ship, which included the words: 'FEMALE KARYOTYPE 46XX'. The forty-six referred to the number of chromosomes – the normal number for human beings – and the XX referred to the presence of two X chromosomes, which meant that Lesley Brown's child was to be a girl.

Arousing interest

The Browns made frequent visits from Bristol to Oldham, and these visits soon aroused suspicion, among those not directly involved, that she was pregnant. When the couple went to Oldham, they would stay in secret locations, and they used a code word when they telephoned the hospital. Despite the secrecy, word got out to the press, some members of which went to enormous lengths to find out whatever details they could about the case. Some dressed as hospital porters or window cleaners. Large sums of money were offered for the slightest piece of information. In Bristol, reporters waited eagerly outside the Browns' house. A nurse remembers the interest of the press: 'You were stopped in the street because you worked at Oldham. It didn't matter whether you were a cleaner or what you were, but you worked at Oldham and you were asked: did you know anything about this, did you know anything about that.'

Just over six weeks before the end of her pregnancy, in June 1978, Lesley Brown was admitted to the maternity ward at the Oldham General Hospital, under an assumed name. One of the nurses remembers: 'Believe it or not she was in the day room on the maternity unit. A vast room: but you couldn't see a wall, you couldn't see anything – it was just cards, flowers, it was just a huge room of pink.' As late as one month before delivery, the baby's weight was considerably lower than average. However, she began to develop more rapidly, and when she was born her weight was a healthy 5lb 12oz (2.7kg).

As the day of the birth drew nearer, the pressure on the Browns, and on Steptoe, was enormous. There was even a bomb scare, presumably a hoax to root out Lesley Brown for photographs and a good story. Steptoe took Mrs Brown in a wheelchair – with a shawl over her head to cover her face if necessary – through the basement to another part of the hospital. The building was searched, but no explosives were found. Perhaps the most upsetting example of press intrusion was the report in a local paper that Lesley Brown's baby was about to die. The Browns were understandably very distressed, and Steptoe did all he could to reassure them that all signs indicated that the baby would be healthy.

By the later stages of the pregnancy, Lesley Brown was convinced that everything would go smoothly: 'I wouldn't do any knitting earlier on because although I thought I was pregnant I didn't want to ruin everything. I didn't want to push my luck and we wouldn't buy baby stuff or anything like that.'

The birth of an idea
On 25 July 1978, Steptoe decided that the birth should go ahead. Tests had indicated that the baby could be delivered safely. Lesley Brown's toxaemia meant that a normal birth could have complications, and so it was decided to deliver the baby by caesarean section. With utmost secrecy, Steptoe rallied the relevant people, and made sure that Lesley Brown did not eat or drink anything. Much of the preparation for the birth was carried out under torch light, as the press watching the third-floor window would have been suspicious if the lights had been turned on. A film crew from the Central Office of Information was to record the historic birth. Everything was made ready, and at 11.31pm anaesthetic and muscle relaxant were administered to the expectant mother. At 11.38, she was wheeled into the operating theatre, and at 11.42, Steptoe made the first incision. John Webster remembers that moment:

'People from the Central Office of Information were there, and of course they had a massive crew in those days. Paediatricians were there, and other people who'd been involved with the work. Everybody wanted to be in on the final act. I'll always remember Patrick making the first incision, and just keeping my fingers crossed – not literally, because I was assisting him. I was hoping that everything would turn out all right and hoping that Louise would come out perfectly normal. And she did.'

The baby was lifted clear of Lesley Brown's womb at 11.47; she took a deep breath, then began to cry loudly. Steptoe made a point of showing Lesley Brown's womb to the cameras – the total lack of fallopian tubes proved that this was no ordinary baby. After Steptoe finished the surgery, Edwards and Purdy joined him in the theatre.

John Brown had been waiting in Lesley's hospital room. One of the nurses was given the happy duty of informing him that the operation had been a success: 'You may go and see your baby daughter now,' she said. John Brown ran to the operating theatre, and was handed his new daughter:

> 'When this nurse actually passed [Louise] to me. . . I'm looking at her, and I was trembling, shaking, and I thought, this is a miracle. That's the thing that sticks in my mind: when I had her in my arms, for the very first time.'

The birth was announced at a press conference held at Prestwich Hospital, and Edwards and Steptoe gave interviews to television crews. Steptoe later recalled, in his own account of the birth: 'It was Bob's brain, skill and perseverance and Jean's hard working devotion which led to this wonderful moment of achievement.'

Chapter 5

IVF EXPLOSION

'For two or three years it was wonderful, and the ethical ride was straightforward; people understood at last what we were trying to do... I remember that when Louise Brown went home with her mum and dad, the neighbours welcomed her with a street party.'

Robert Edwards

The first few years after the momentous, highly publicized birth of Louise Brown in July 1978 were indeed a time of fairly unfettered experimentation in the field of IVF.

In the months after the birth, the experimental programme at Kershaw's Cottage Hospital quickly wound down. Patrick Steptoe had been due to retire in June 1978, but had stayed on to the end of Lesley Brown's pregnancy. So now his days working for the National Health Service were over. There were three more healthy pregnancies under way at Kershaw's. Two were lost: one of them rejected by the patient's body as the embryo had a chromosomal abnormality, and the other tragically miscarried five months into the pregnancy, while its mother was fell-walking in Yorkshire. The other pregnancy did go to term, and the world's second 'test-tube baby', Alistair Montgomery, was delivered in Glasgow in January 1979. This confirmed to the world that the birth of Louise Brown six months before was not a fluke: it proved that IVF really worked. Suddenly, there was hope for many of the millions of infertile couples all over the world. In 1980, Robert Edwards and Patrick Steptoe set up the world's first private IVF clinic – Bourn Hall, near Cambridge – and they began taking patients from around the world. Edwards recalls:

'We had a wonderful team of young people, including Simon Fishel, Jacques Cohen, Carol Veheely and others, wonderful young people, keen as mustard they were, loving their work, loving the way they were helping their patients, and some very fine young doctors – it was a fantastic team.'

Lacking National Health Service funding, they raised the money from other sources. They had one major financial backer at the outset, who bought the building and helped to set up temporary wards. But the sponsors withdrew from the deal. Muriel Harris, who had been a key member of the team in Oldham and helped Edwards and Steptoe to set up the clinic, remembers why the financial support was withdrawn:

'They were worried about litigation if anything went wrong. They were perfectly happy until they discovered that we were going to treat American patients and I think that was just the final straw: the enormous payments in litigation that could be commanded in American courts was just not worth the risk.'

Edwards, Steptoe and the team set up their wards and an operating theatre in Portakabins in the grounds of Bourn Hall. Edwards sets the scene:

'We had to take hold of the whole of this field and make it work. We had to look at. . . embryo growth, embryo culture, chromosomes; we had to know about embryos, about fertilization, we had to know about the ovaries, about the follicles – how they grew, how we'd stimulate them – we had to know about patients; if our transfer techniques were wrong, if they could be improved. . . We had to have trained nurses, trained counsellors, we had to have an ethical committee, we had to set up all of these organizations with very little experience . . . Before we had the first patient in, all our systems had to be tested and proved. I think we used mouse embryos to test our system. . . so many groups were now start-ing, even before we'd opened Bourn Hall. The delay of two and a half years was now proving a very heavy burden on us, because you had to pick up everything again . . . and we did, we got started.'

The first IVF baby outside the UK was Candice Reed, born in Australia on 23 June 1980. The first American IVF baby followed quickly: Elizabeth Carr was conceived at a centre run by Edwards's old friends, Howard and Georgeanna Jones – the first American IVF clinic – in Norfolk, Virginia.

Proceeding with caution
Despite all the new centres and the positive press that IVF began to attract, and the hope that it gave to infertile couples, it was still subject to caution and ethical debate. One of the main ethical concerns in the early days of IVF was the possibility of creating 'monsters'. The birth of four healthy babies produced by IVF was, quite rightly, not enough to convince everyone that IVF is totally safe. What if IVF babies develop abnormally as they grow older, or one in ten is severely abnormal?

In the late 1970s, Edwards himself proposed an international follow-up study of the progress of children who had been conceived by IVF, but an advisory group for the Medical Research Council (MRC) decided against the idea, on the grounds that it would make IVF children feel different from normal children. However, some such studies do exist. In the UK in 1983 the London School of Hygiene and Tropical Medicine set up a national register of IVF births, partly funded by money from the MRC. And the National Perinatal Statistics Unit in Sydney, Australia, has produced comprehensive statistics on IVF babies since the late 1970s. Their data actually suggest that IVF children are slightly smaller, more premature and more likely to develop birth defects, in particular spina bifida and abnormalities of the heart than non-IVF babies. This is likely to be due to the rate of multiple pregnancies, which is higher than for normal conception, rather than any damage sustained by the chromosomes during IVF. This reinforces the reason for the rule, adopted in many countries, that no more than three embryos should be transferred in any one cycle, to reduce the numbers of multiple pregnancies. Having said this, IVF babies have more or less the same chances of being normal and healthy as do children conceived in the natural way. There are many thousands of happy, healthy human beings around the world, who would not be here if it were not for IVF, who would testify to its positive effects.

The other main ethical issue relating to IVF remains hotly debated to this day. It is the fact that IVF involves experimentation with embryos. Some people consider human embryos to be human individuals, while others see them just as clumps of cells, with no identity. Some of those who hold the first point of view equate the destruction of human embryos with abortion or murder: an embryo cannot give its consent to its destruction, just as a foetus does not choose to be aborted. Cases in which the embryo being destroyed was created purely for research are considered by some to be worse than abortion. Even those who do not share this view are well aware that experiments on embryos are more likely to require exhaustive ethical consideration than many other areas of medical science. On the other hand, some argued that abortion had become legal (in 1967 in the UK), so why should there be restrictions on destruction of an embryo, which is at a much earlier stage of development? What made matters more ironic for these people was that abortions could be paid for by the state – through the National Health Service – while no funding was available for IVF. In any case, the ethical wrangles continued, but IVF practice gathered momentum into the 1980s.

During the five years after the birth of Louise Brown, IVF clinics were set up in many countries, including Israel and Singapore and several in Europe as well as those in Australia and the USA. IVF found no state funding in the United Kingdom, and so research had been effectively stalled. Teams outside the UK which had been in competition with Edwards and Steptoe to achieve the first baby born by IVF now forged ahead with new experimental techniques. Some of these techniques are now part of routine IVF practice, but at the time were daring ventures into the unknown. The most significant centre of research at the time was Monash University in Melbourne, Australia.

Getting the team together
The key members of the IVF team in Melbourne were Edwin Carlyle (Carl) Wood and Alan Trounson. During the late 1960s, Wood had developed an artificial fallopian tube, which he hoped would cure the infertility of women whose tubes were blocked – just as IVF had attempted to do (and eventually succeeded). Wood tested the tube in pigs, but it did not work. At a conference in 1970, where Wood presented a paper on his artificial tube, another reproductive biologist, Neil Moore, suggested that Wood could try embryo transfer to overcome infertility. Moore had been working on sheep: prize ewes were given fertility drugs and then artificially inseminated. The many embryos produced were taken from those ewes, and carried to term by other, less valuable ones. On a typical day, he would transfer hundreds of embryos. Wood was aware of the work being carried out by Edwards and Steptoe on the other side of the world, and decided to take Moore's advice. In the meantime, Wood attempted to carry out a variation of Moore's work, in humans. He wanted to transfer an embryo from a fertile woman 'donor' to an infertile woman but, with everything ready to go, the prospective donor fell

pregnant too early. Wood realized that IVF offered a better solution for infertile patients anyway, as the babies produced by the technique would be genetically related to the parents.

Moore was important in the story in another way: he was supervising Alan Trounson at the time, and he suggested that Trounson join Wood's team. At first, Trounson was not interested in working on human IVF. Instead, he went to carry out research into freezing cattle embryos, at Cambridge University in the UK. He remained there until 1976. When Trounson joined the Melbourne team in 1977, IVF research was already well under way. Trounson brought to the team his expertise in animals. He saw human IVF as a refinement of IVF in animals: he jokes that, in terms of fertility treatment, 'a woman is just an upright sheep'. Also on the team were gynaecologist John Leeton; Alex Lapata, a Polish biologist; and Ian Johnston, who had heard Edwards speak at the Tokyo symposium in 1971. Johnston left the team in 1980, to set up his own IVF team, also in Melbourne.

Wood and his colleagues were to stride ahead in new IVF techniques, and they achieved an impressive list of firsts. Wood explains:

'We were in a hurry because we had a good team. We were going well. We wanted to do everything, and we wanted to do it as quickly as possible – because there were certainly a lot of opponents to our work and we didn't know when the lobby against us might persuade the government or some other hospital bodies to oppose and stop our work.'

Super ovulation down-under

The Melbourne team had been in competition with Edwards and Steptoe since the early 1970s, and at last found their first success in 1980: the birth of Candice Reed. They had about eight pregnancies in that year, but the success rate was still very low. The team decided to use the fertility drug clomiphene to stimulate the production of several eggs at the same time in women's ovaries. Edwards and Steptoe had tried this technique, but the hormones had adversely affected the whole of the menstrual cycle: although they were collecting many eggs from each woman, those eggs, once fertilized, would not implant properly. Some members of the team in Melbourne had extensive experience with the use of fertility drugs in domestic animals, and worked out the best ways to use them to control women's cycles. Soon they began to produce larger numbers

of eggs, and began to increase their success rates by transferring
more than one egg at a time. Trounson recalls:

'The trouble was, women ovulate all hours of the day and some terribly
inappropriate times at night, like two or three in the morning, or four
or five in the morning. So you're getting everybody up to collect a
single egg from a single follicle. I realized it was a mug's game. . . I went
to Carl and said, "Look, this is nuts. I mean, I've been trained in
reproductive biology: I know how to superovulate animals. This has
got to work because it works for all the animals that I've ever worked
with." And I said: "Will you give us some patients?" . . . And of course
they turned out to be the initial studies that got us a whole run of
pregnancies, because instead of going in there to collect one egg from
one follicle we were usually collecting eggs from three or four follicles.
So we had two or three or four eggs to work with.'

The regime of hormone drugs used to induce superovulation and
control the female patients' menstrual cycles forms the basis of
hormone treatments used in modern IVF. Typically a dozen eggs,
but as many as thirty, are collected at one time from a woman undergoing these treatments. Incidentally, some women who are infertile
due to low egg production are sometimes given these hormones, as
'fertility drugs'. The use of fertility drugs – often synthetic hormones
– began in the 1960s. They induce the women to superovulate,
increasing the chance of eggs being produced, and hopefully
fertilized. At present, this is an inexact science, and in some cases the
woman involved produces several eggs, more than one of which
may be fertilized. This has led, in the last four decades, to unusual
multiple births, which have often captured media attention. The case
of Mandy Allwood, for example, hit the headlines in 1996 when she
became pregnant with eight foetuses after a course of fertility drugs.
These potential octuplets – none of whom survived – were not
identical: each foetus had grown from a different embryo, which
arose from the fertilization of a different egg. It is extremely rare for
a natural pregnancy to have more than two non-identical foetuses.
This is simply because, during most months, a fertile woman
produces just one egg. Fertility drugs increase the frequency of
multiple births because they induce women to produce more than
one egg per cycle. The twins, triplets, quads and so on produced as a
result of fertility drugs are mostly non-identical, since they come
from several separate eggs. The twins or triplets in multiple

pregnancies produced by IVF are likewise mostly non-identical, because they result from the transfer of two or three embryos. Identical twins are the result of an embryo breaking into two or more fragments, each one of which implants and grows to become a separate individual. It seems that this is as common in nature as it is in IVF or with fertility drugs.

The introduction of superovulation improved the Melbourne team's success rate dramatically. One consequence of this approach was that many more embryos were produced than could be implanted safely in one go. Initially, 'spare' embryos were discarded, but later the team decided to adopt a new strategy: they would freeze the left-over embryos in liquid nitrogen (at minus 196 degrees Celsius); then, if the first attempt failed, frozen embryos would be thawed and transferred in a new attempt.

Freezing and thawing

Edwards had tried to freeze and subsequently thaw embryos in 1977, but for a different reason: he wanted to delay the transfer of the embryos until the most suitable time during the female patients' menstrual cycles. But he had no success: the embryos he froze did not continue to develop once they had been thawed. Alan Trounson had worked on freezing cattle embryos at Cambridge University in the UK, and he applied his expertise to the freezing of human embryos. Carl Wood recalls some of the thoughts and feelings around the time that his team introduced this technique, called cryopreservation: in particular the development of the ethical stance taken by the hospital at which he was working:

> 'The results of embryo freezing – as far as the offspring were concerned – in cattle and certainly in sheep were not adverse, there was no harmful effect to freezing or thawing an embryo if it survived that procedure. Only two out of three embryos survived the process and some people have thought that the freeze—thawing is in some ways a test of its normality or its robustness and that's why there's not going to be any risk to do freezing and thawing. . . We sat down with an ethics committee, a group of ethics people at the Queen Victoria Hospital in Melbourne, to discuss our problem and the suggestion of embryo freezing. Our own Catholic moral theologian didn't agree with IVF, and he also thought he didn't really agree with freezing. But he thought freezing was better than discarding the embryos.'

Like hormone treatments designed to induce superovulation, cryopreservation has become standard procedure in most IVF clinics. The role played by cryopreservation has been turned on its head: rather than solving the problem of spare embryos, as the technique was originally developed to do, cryopreservation now enables IVF clinics to produce spare embryos purposefully, with significant benefits to the patients. For example, as many as thirty eggs can be collected from a woman in a single operation, and most or all of them may be fertilized. If the first embryo transfer is unsuccessful, the woman can return each subsequent month until pregnancy is achieved, and two or three embryos may be thawed prior to each visit. This greatly reduces the physical and emotional stress on patients undergoing IVF treatment, and makes the cost of continuing the treatment much less prohibitive: a large part of the financial burden of IVF treatment is contained within the initial stages, in particular egg retrieval.

Cryopreservation allows each couple to have a reserve of embryos that can be thawed and transferred relatively cheaply and easily. Another benefit of freezing embryos applies to couples where one or both partners are undergoing treatment that may result in future infertility. Chemotherapy, used to eradicate cancer, is perhaps the best example. When the woman is no longer producing eggs, or the man is no longer producing sperm, the embryos can be transferred to the woman's womb, where they may implant and bring about a pregnancy which would not have been possible without cryo-preservation. More on this in Chapters 9 and 10. Similarly, a woman may want to delay having children, even if she is not undergoing chemotherapy. For example, a woman may want to have her first child in her forties, when she has achieved other life goals. Normally, this would increase the likelihood of genetic abnormalities such as those that lead to Down syndrome. Cryopreservation offers a new possibility for women faced with an exclusive choice of children and career. Now, in principle at least, they can have both, without the increased chance of their children having genetic diseases.

The use of cryopreservation to this end is the subject of some debate: some people think it is tampering with nature just too much, and for selfish reasons, or that there may be other, unforeseen dangers in enabling older women to carry a pregnancy to term. In any case, embryos are routinely frozen now, for a variety of reasons, and no ill effects have been suffered by the children born from frozen–thawed embryos.

How does it work?

Freezing normally destroys a living cell. The main reason for this concerns the cell's water content. A typical cell is up to 80 per cent water and, as water freezes, it forms ice crystals that take up more space than the liquid water. In the same way as ice can burst water pipes during cold weather, the water inside a cell expands as it freezes, forming ice that ruptures the cell membrane. Incidentally, this is the cause of frostbite: tissues of the extremities, such as the skin of fingers, receive a reduced blood supply in very cold weather, as the body tries to lessen its heat loss. The cells of these tissues quickly cool, then freeze, rupture and die. If this happens to the cells that make up an embryo, the embryo will not continue to grow once it has thawed. So, how is this problem overcome?

The key lies in dehydration: the water is actually removed from the cells that make up the embryo. Embryos to be frozen are kept in small plastic straws or glass vials, which are then immersed in saline solution (salty water). The temperature of the solution is very slowly reduced – by about 1 degree Celsius every three minutes – and the solution surrounding the cells begins to freeze. As it does, the solution contains less and less water: and so the concentration of salt in the saline solution increases. This causes water to 'leak out' through each cell's membrane. The process by which water passes through a membrane between two solutions at different concentrations is called osmosis. It is responsible for water being 'sucked up' from soil into the roots of a plant. The 'osmotic pressure' in this case is enough to push water up to the top of the tallest trees. Water is taken slowly from inside an embryonic cell by osmosis, so that the cell cannot rupture as its temperature drops. Once the temperature of the whole mixture has dropped to well below freezing, it is plunged into liquid nitrogen. Substances called cryoprotectants – which act in the same way as antifreeze in a motor car engine – are mixed in with the saline solution just before freezing. They help to ensure that the water in the solution freezes at a temperature lower than the normal freezing point, as well as protecting the cell from physical damage during freezing and thawing. When an embryo is cooled to a very low temperature, metabolic activity inside its cells effectively stops, and the cells do not age. The embryo can be kept in 'suspended animation' for perhaps hundreds of years.

The thawing process is not always as slow or precise as the freezing. In some cases, the frozen embryos – still in their straws or glass vials – are simply plunged into warm water, at body temperature. Whether rapid or slow and controlled, this warming unfreezes the water in the solution surrounding the embryos, and rehydrates the embryos' cells. Rarely do all the cells that make up an embryo survive, but it was shown in animals that embryos that suffer even substantial damage during cryopreservation can usually recover and grow.

In many quarters the reaction to the freezing of human embryos was one of horror. One episode sticks in Wood's mind:

'We had a young Roman Catholic priest who sat in the central square of Melbourne, who said he'd fast to death until we promised not to freeze any more embryos. . . Alan was overseas at the time. . . I sent him a message: I said, "Alan, would you mind coming down to the square and fasting with this guy to sort of put in a protest in case he's getting too ill." But fortunately we were lucky: the Archbishop in Melbourne persuaded the priest to stop his fast, and things quietened down.'

It was not until 1983 that the team achieved the first pregnancy using a frozen–thawed embryo. The woman involved had received three embryos directly after fertilization and, though these implanted, the pregnancy miscarried after eight weeks. A fourth embryo produced by the initial IVF had been frozen at the eight-cell stage. When it was thawed – some four months after fertilization had taken place – it was found that two of the eight cells had, in fact, ruptured. Animal studies had shown that the chances were good that the embryo would recover despite having two ruptured cells. The thawed embryo did implant normally, and developed to twenty-four weeks, before, sadly, it too miscarried.

'Ice babies'

The outcry over embryo freezing was quelled to a certain extent by the birth of Zoe Leyland, on 11 April 1984. Zoe's mother, Loretta, recalls:

'Professor Leeton came to see me in hospital after I had eleven eggs, and said I had a couple of options. One was to freeze the embryos. It was something new, and it just seemed natural to give that a go and that's what we did.'

Zoe was the first baby produced by the Melbourne team from a frozen–thawed embryo: and the term 'ice baby' came into popular parlance, just as 'test-tube baby' had done some years earlier. A newspaper in Australia featured a big photograph of the moment of birth, focusing on the baby's head: the first time a photograph like this had been featured. IVF was big news once again. Carl Wood admires the courage of Zoe's parents:

> 'Oh, I think they were very brave. I think all those couples in the seventies and early eighties were very brave because we hadn't delivered several hundred babies from IVF. And I didn't really relax completely until about 500 babies were born.'

Zoe wasn't the very first 'ice baby'. In fact the first birth from a frozen–thawed embryo had been in December 1983, in Holland – and it was twins. The first babies produced from frozen–thawed embryos in Britain originated at Bourn Hall. Jacques Cohen, one of the team there, remembers the early days of freezing. He was appointed by Edwards largely because of his experience with freezing embryos. Cohen began by using a substance called glycerol, as a kind of 'anti-freeze':

> 'There was a paper coming out in the journal *Nature* from the Australian group where they had used early embryos and used another anti-freeze... It was done by the Australians; it had a very clear purpose; it meant that you didn't throw extra embryos away. It was a very ethical technique actually: you preserve embryos for later use. So once that happened I think Patrick and Bob decided: "Others have done it, we can now do it," and we went ahead and did it.'

The first such baby in the UK was Gregory Jackson. His father Tony remembers:

> '... tears trickling down my cheeks, you know, we've cracked it. Gregory was there, he was born, he was in front of us. I remember Janet trembling and then being handed Gregory. Yeah, it was really special. Wonderful. Words are not going to help; it's all the feelings that run through you, all happening there: you'd achieved your goal.'

New directions
The work of the Melbourne team during the frenetic period of IVF research in the early 1980s greatly increased the success rate of IVF, and laid the foundation of standard practice in the field. The only

notable exceptions are the development of ultrasound-guided egg collection, by Susan Lenz and Matts Wickland in Scandinavia; intracytoplasmic sperm injection (ICSI), developed in Belgium, which makes it possible to treat the infertile man by IVF; and the development of 'GnRH analogs' (chemicals that mimic the action of a natural hormone to help control superovulation) in Scotland.

Meanwhile, in England, research into IVF was picking up again, and new centres were opening. There was the Humana Hospital, run by Ian Craft, and the IVF centre at Hammersmith Hospital, run by Robert Winston. Both of these centres are in London. With limited state funding, Craft's team produced the first IVF twins on the National Heath Service – IVF was no longer exclusively for the rich, although even now all but about 18 per cent of IVF is provided by the private sector. Winston, a former opponent of IVF, was to become one of the most publicly recognized advocates of IVF.

In January 1984, the team in Melbourne achieved another first: a baby produced by embryo donation. As with much of the pioneering work in Melbourne, Alan Trounson had carried out this procedure with animals, and felt sure that it would work with humans. It is interesting to note that a child produced by embryo donation is not genetically related to either its 'father' or 'mother'.

Perhaps the most interesting part of the story of embryo donation is not the first successful birth, but the events surrounding the first pregnancy, achieved in the previous year. This caused a row between the UK (Edwards and Steptoe) and Australia (Wood and Trounson). The donated embryo was produced by fertilizing an egg – with sperm from an anonymous donor – that had come from a patient who was receiving IVF treatment. It was given to another woman on the IVF programme. (Her husband was infertile, and there were risks involved with collecting eggs from her own ovaries.) The embryo was transferred, and implanted in the recipient's womb. Unfortunately, this first ever pregnancy involving a donated embryo was to end with miscarriage ten weeks later. Edwards's and Steptoe's main objection concerned the age of the egg donor: she was forty-two. As noted earlier, women of this age are more likely than average to produce foetuses with abnormalities. The response from the Melbourne team was that the recipient was aware of the risks, and had decided for herself to go ahead, as no other embryos were available at the time. In a letter to the *British Medical Journal*, Edwards and Steptoe suggested that 'strict ethical guidelines' should be drawn up. The arguments over this case have long since disappeared, but the fact that there was major disagreement between the two most important IVF teams illustrates how rapid the progress of the Melbourne team was: so rapid that even Edwards and Steptoe – normally fighting for, rather than against, new procedures – objected to it. As Trounson says:

'These kinds of things get reported in the media as yet another world first, which starts to raise the political pressures here; because "God, what are they going to do next? We've got to get a law and make sure that we're in control of this." So in Victoria [Australia], the world's first legislation appears. And it was the Infertility Procedures Act: the first piece of legislature in this area in the world.'

Exerting some control

This was indeed the first actual legislation in the field of IVF, but ethical guidelines already existed – in Australia, the UK and elsewhere. Prior to the birth of Louise Brown in 1978, many ethical discussions – both formal and informal – had taken place regarding the ethics of IVF in general and embryo research in particular, and some guidelines were already in place. In 1978, the British Medical Research Council set up an advisory group to review policies relating to IVF and embryo research. The group decided that embryo research could be carried out as long as it had clear scientific aims. It saw IVF as a therapeutic procedure, which should be subject to the same ethical considerations as the normal doctor—patient relationship. In 1979, the Ethics Advisory Board of the United States Department of Health, Education and Welfare published a report: 'Support of Research Involving Human *in vitro* Fertilization and Embryo Transfer'. One of its key conclusions was: 'No embryos will be sustained *in vitro* beyond the stage normally associated with implantation (fourteen days after fertilization)'. Like the British group, the US Department of Health suggested that research would be allowed if that research had clear scientific or medical goals. In 1982, the National Health and Medical Research Council in Australia put together a similar report. It recognized the fact that research on embryos, eggs and sperm was necessary to the continued development of IVF, but again with certain conditions. A working group at the British Medical Association made a report in the *British Medical Journal*, in May 1983, with conclusions along the same lines.

These ethical debates were set in the scientific and medical circles, not in government. Legislation on IVF and embryo research – including in some countries the formation of regulatory and licensing bodies – would come later.

Superovulation and cryopreservation brought with them new challenges for the scientists, medical professionals and politicians involved in IVF. One of the most famous, or perhaps infamous, cases involved 'orphaned embryos'. A couple from Los Angeles, Mario and Elsa Rios, received IVF treatment from Carl Wood and his team in Melbourne, in June 1981. Wood himself takes up the story:

'I got a call I think at two in the morning from a writer from London: someone working on one of the newspapers there, wanting to interview me about the Rioses' embryos. He said. . . there are some embryos that you're involved with in Melbourne. . . and the parents of the embryos have died in an aeroplane accident. . . I suddenly realized that it was the Rios couple, who'd come to us from Los Angeles, because at that stage on the west coast [of America] there was little or no IVF. . . They went through several IVF treatments in Melbourne and I think on the second one they had some embryos frozen, I did a fresh embryo transfer. It didn't work. . . I waited until the morning just to check all the records. No one knew what to do with the frozen embryos because. . . there were hardly any relatives available. . .'

It turned out that the Rioses were very rich, and – with no other heirs – the embryos suddenly became heirs to a huge fortune. Large numbers of women volunteered to carry the embryos to term: as surrogate mothers for the dead couple. No doubt the possible financial gains had something to do with that – indeed, when American and Australian authorities decided that the embryos had no claim to the Rioses' fortune, the flood of surrogacy offers diminished considerably. With no conclusive decision on the fate of the embryos, they have remained in liquid nitrogen, in a tank in the Queen Victoria Medical Centre, ever since. If the Rioses' embryos were to be thawed, it is unlikely that they would develop normally, as they were frozen in the early days of cryopreservation, when the technique had not been perfected.

Some of the advances in IVF ultimately resulted in the destruction of hundreds of embryos, and this began to attract the attention of members of religious communities, anti-abortionists and politicians. Could it be right that a cure for infertility necessitates the large-scale destruction of human embryos? Many saw the experiments with

human life as no different from the immoral human experiments carried out in the German concentration camps during World War II, in particular by Dr Mengele. Also known as the Angel of Death, Mengele carried out experiments on prisoners of war and inmates of concentration camps. Some of his experiments aimed to discover ways of increasing fertility, to benefit the German race.
Alan Trounson recalls:

'There were walls daubed with whitewash about "Wood and Trounson: mass murderers", and newspaper articles which were highly offensive. And even television programmes run – one of them by the BBC – which interposed us with Mengele and the experiments of Nazi Germany. So, yes, there was a lot of criticism.'

In 1984, Robert Edwards was effectively charged with murder. The charge was brought, under the 1861 Offences Against the Person Act, by *Life News*, published by the anti-abortion organization LIFE. Edwards's reaction:

'I read an article in *The Times*, and that's all I knew. And then I asked my lawyer what would happen, and he said it will go nowhere because there's no law in that field. And so we waited, and that was the decision that the Director of Public Prosecutions gave. So it never bothered us to any great extent. You must realize that we knew that many people were objecting to what we were doing: several popes objected, so we knew it was a field of great controversy.'

Embryo research throws up serious moral as well as ethical issues. Many people do object publicly to it. In the words of Nuala Scarisbrick, campaigner for LIFE:

'It is wrong deliberately to manufacture human beings in laboratories. It's particularly wrong to manufacture more than you can reasonably use. The dilemmas of what to do with spare embryos were not faced up by those creating them. There was no regulation. I think there still is very little regulation. The human misery of childlessness, I began to feel early in the eighties, was being used as a kind of cover for a runaway research and experimentation upon completely vulnerable human beings: namely, the pre-born person. And it's a leap for anybody to see something no bigger than a full stop – the newly created embryo – as a real human person. But I got to understand that early on, and we now know, through all the amazing information that genetics has produced, that actually each one of us is there at the moment of fertilization. We are genetically complete then.'

Chapter 6

Whose life is it anyway?

'A society which had no inhibiting limits, especially in the areas with which we have been concerned, questions of birth and death, of the setting up of families, and the valuing of human life, would be a society without moral scruples. *And this nobody wants.*'

The Committee of Inquiry into Human Fertilization and Embryology, 1984

During the 1970s, the ethical and moral debates surrounding IVF and embryo research had been largely confined to the scientific community and the media. Medical research organizations in several countries set up ethical committees, and newspapers, radio and television considered some of the consequences of IVF. But no laws were passed. During the 1980s, however, the debates began to spread to the political arena. The result of this was legislation that created the world's first IVF regulatory body: the Human Fertilization and Embryology Authority (HFEA), in the UK. The legislation was called the Human Fertilization and Embryology Act, and was passed in 1990. It was only the second piece of legislation ever passed concerning IVF and embryology: in 1984, in Australia, the Infertility Procedures Act was passed by the government of the State of Victoria.

Embryo research: right or wrong?
For most of us, the idea of experimenting with human embryos is at least profound. Embryos are tiny pieces of human life. They are fundamental and perplexing. So it is not surprising that there exists a continuum of opinions about IVF and human embryo research. At one extreme of this continuum are those who would welcome a situation in which there was no regulation at all. This would give scientists a free rein to carry out whatever research they wanted to,

without reference to collective moral judgement and ethical codes. However, this could enable some individuals to carry out the most undesirable studies, resulting in human suffering rather than the alleviation of infertility or the eradication of disabling genetic diseases. But, some would argue, such individuals will carry out their work, in secret if necessary, whether the law permits them to or not. Specific restrictions could mean that a particular piece of potentially useful research cannot be carried out, because of a rule of law that may be in effect quite arbitrary. For example, the fourteen-day limit on keeping embryos alive outside the body, enforced by law in many countries, is actually fairly arbitrary. Yet it means, for example, that research which could benefit from experiments with a sixteen-day-old embryo is illegal.

At the other end of the continuum of opinion are those who believe firmly that all IVF and all embryo research is wholly unnatural and immoral; that both should be outlawed, on moral grounds. Many – but not all – of these people arrive at this point of view from spiritual or religious considerations. The term 'ensoulment' is sometimes used to describe the process by which an embryo becomes a person: a human individual. The relevance of this to embryo research is clearly a matter of belief: if ensoulment happens, then surely it is immoral to carry out experiments on human embryos. Many religious thinkers condemn IVF as immoral, too. The Vatican, for example, considers it wrong in principle, and against God's will, to remove the sexual act from the baby-making process.

Not everyone is so extremely for or against embryo research. Those who are to be found around the middle of the continuum – who are perhaps in the majority – are happy with the kind of regulation that is facilitated by the HFEA, including sanctioning human embryo research if it has clear, clinical aims. These varied opinions conflict with one another, and people who hold differing beliefs often find themselves at loggerheads with each other. In certain contexts – such as in government – this conflict of opinion can lead to bitter debate.

In the early 1980s, these concerns over embryo research were focused on two new IVF procedures: superovulation and cryopreservation, described in Chapter 5. Superovulation ultimately resulted in the death of many embryos – those that were not implanted – while cryopreservation was seen by some as inhumane. In 1982 an ITV programme was screened, featuring Robert Edwards and Patrick Steptoe at their Bourn Hall clinic, discussing how they stored frozen embryos. On the same programme was Michael Thomas, head of the ethics committee for the British Medical Association, calling for a moratorium on human embryo research, as he recalls:

'We hadn't discussed it: we hadn't looked at the social implications, we hadn't looked at the moral implications, and we hadn't looked at the financial implications. And I was calling for a pause: let's just break for a moment, let's just think this thing through, don't let's go helter skelter and suddenly find that something that seemed to be a good idea actually wasn't such a good idea in the end.'

Such a break in research would require legislation, and that would have to involve Parliament. A moratorium on research would act like a brake, cautiously applied to prevent reproductive science and technology from going out of control. There would be no moratorium in the UK, and research continued until and after the 1990 Human Fertilization and Embryology Act.

Two types of embryo
Human embryo research involves two distinct types of embryos. First there are 'spare' ones, produced by IVF with the intention of their being transferred into a woman's body. They become spare either because the woman becomes pregnant and no longer needs them, or because the embryos were not viable. Then there are 'research' embryos, again produced by fertilizing eggs outside the body. This time, however, the egg is donated by a woman, purely for research purposes. One of the driving forces behind the call for the moratorium on human embryo research, and therefore the involvement of Government, was the moral revulsion that many felt towards any embryo research – particularly the second kind. Pro-life campaigner Jack Scarisbrick, trustee of LIFE and husband of Nuala, quoted in Chapter 5, recalls:

'When we heard about superovulation, and what had been happening in Australia, the full gravity of the situation became apparent. I remember thinking, "Right, for every one child who is now being produced live, there are dozens who are perishing . . ." Then of course, we heard about freezing and our reaction to that was to say, "A civilized society does not put human beings in the freezer." We now learn that the freezing, or maybe the unfreezing, kills a lot of these young human beings. I think I'm right in saying only about 4 per cent of the human beings who are being manufactured in the laboratories are alive today. The rest are either dead or in the deep freezer.'

The LIFE organization became vociferous public opponents of human embryo research, on moral grounds. They demanded that there should be no multiple fertilization, so that there would be no spare embryos on which to carry out laboratory experimentation. They wanted action as soon as possible. Another highly public figure in the whole IVF debate was Phyllis Bowman, the leader of the pro-life organization the Society for the Protection of the Unborn Child (SPUC). The Society saw IVF as the 'manufacture' of human beings. One feature common to all forms of manufacture, it argued, is quality control. SPUC recognized that quality control, in IVF, meant that 'defective' embryos, which would have produced disabled babies, would be discarded. This kind of 'quality control' has indeed become possible, by testing embryos for genetic abnormalities (see Chapter 7). SPUC believe strongly that disabled people have as much right as anyone to life, and this was one reason they disagreed with IVF. From the time of Louise Brown's birth, throughout the 1980s, Bowman appeared frequently on television campaigning against IVF.

What sort of research was being carried out involving human embryos? Much of it was aimed at improving the then very poor success rates of IVF. Examples of this 'applied' research included work at Cambridge, ironically funded by the Government through the Medical Research Council. It investigated the effects on the embryo of chemical agents called oxygen free radicals. Free radicals are very reactive and can damage the embryo, rendering it unable to develop. They are rare inside the body; but in the air, where oxygen is plentiful, oxygen free radicals are more common. The researchers' experiments aimed to discover the effects of free radicals on a developing embryo, and whether a different culture medium might reduce those effects. Another example of research was an investigation of the effects of temperature on an embryo's delicate internal framework (the cytoskeleton). The temperature inside a woman's body is just over 37 degrees Celsius, but in a laboratory it is much cooler. It would be uncomfortable to work in a laboratory at that temperature, but the research suggested that embryos kept in warm water baths could stand a better chance of developing normally than those kept at room temperature.

In addition to applied research, there was 'pure' research, designed to improve our general understanding of the human embryo. Of course, the fact that this sort of research is not called 'applied' does not mean that the new knowledge it brings will be of no use. It simply means that it is not aimed at solving specific problems. New discoveries about the workings of eggs, sperms and embryos are likely to be of great use in IVF, at least in a general sense, or in the longer term.

Official consideration
However useful pure or applied research using human embryos may have promised to be, there were those – as we have seen – who objected to it strongly and publicly. The battle lines were drawn between the 'pro-lifers' and those who were 'pro-research'. So in 1982 the Government set up the Committee of Inquiry into Human Fertilization and Embryology. The Committee was headed by Dame Mary Warnock, who recalls that it was the initiative of Norman Fowler, then Secretary of State for Health:

> 'I think [Norman Fowler] wanted a committee because he quite rightly thought that this was a case where legislation would have to brought in. Because in this area people always say, "What's going to happen next? Where's it going to lead? Where's it going to end? Isn't this the slippery slope?" And I think he and his colleagues realized that there were a lot of questions about which people would be very uneasy. But on the other hand, he was terribly unwilling – understandably again – to simply introduce legislation as the result of civil servants drawing up some draft bills. And I think it was a very good case for having either a Royal Commission or – as he had – a Committee of Inquiry.'

The Committee consulted over 200 individuals and organizations during the course of its two-year deliberation, and published its report in July 1984. Dame Mary Warnock, who had worked on several other parliamentary committees, is a philosopher. The other fifteen members of the Committee included representatives of religious communities, legal and medical experts, a social worker, the chair of an area health authority, and psychologists. The Committee's Inquiry was established with the following terms of reference:

> 'To consider recent and potential developments in medicine and science related to human fertilization and embryology; to consider

what policies and safeguards should be applied, including consideration of the social, ethical and legal implications of these developments;
and to make recommendations.'

The Report made a total of sixty-four recommendations, on a variety
of topics including artificial insemination; donation of eggs, sperm
and embryos; surrogacy; and of course IVF and embryo research.
The first, and most important, recommendation suggested that: 'A
new statutory licensing authority be established to regulate both
research and those infertility services which we recommend should
be subject to control.'

Early on, the members of the Committee decided to use the term
'assisted conception' to refer to the various methods of overcoming
infertility. Another term used by some people at the time was
'artificial conception'. The Committee's members agreed that since
the babies produced by these procedures are not artificial, that term
would not be appropriate. There was a general consensus in much of
the discussion that went on between members of the Committee, and
most of the recommendations were supported by all of them.
However, there were some fundamental issues that divided the
Committee, and three statements of dissent were appended to
the report.

One statement concerned surrogate motherhood, while the other
two concerned embryo research. This split of opinion – over embryo
research in particular – extended well beyond the Committee.
Staunch supporters of human embryo research included, of course,
reproductive biologists (scientists who study reproduction) who
were themselves involved in such research. They believed their work
was necessary – either regulated or unregulated – if the success rate
and the safety of IVF was to be improved; or if ways were to be found
of ensuring that children brought into the world as a result of IVF
were as healthy as possible. Without embryo research, scientists
would effectively be researching on the female patients. These
scientists did not want to be prevented from carrying out their work,
and many MPs and other public figures supported them. Others
were horrified by what the scientists were doing with human
embryos, and wanted to make sure that what they saw as immoral
experiments would no longer be permitted. These campaigners, too,
had their supporters within Parliament. The horror these people felt
stemmed from the fact that human embryo research necessitates
carrying out experiments with human beings – or at least potential

human beings. Worse, in by far the majority of cases embryos used in research will perish. Incidentally, this is the main reason that pro-life and anti-abortion campaigners were among those who wanted to see embryo research banned. All embryos are human and alive, of that there is no doubt. On first reckoning, then, it would seem that human embryo research involves carrying out experiments on living human beings. For some, this is enough to call a halt to such research. However, for others, the issue is not quite so straightforward.

An early embryo – at least before any of its cells have become nerve cells (by the process of differentiation, explained in Chapter 1) – cannot feel pain, and is certainly not aware of experiments being performed upon it. However the objections to embryo research are more philosophical and spiritual than scientific. The issue really boils down to: 'Should an embryo, as a potential human being, have the same moral status as an actual human being?' One of the statements of dissent against the majority opinion in the Warnock Report argued that:

'The embryo has a special status because of its potential for development to a stage at which everyone would accord it the status of a human person. It is in our view wrong to create something with the potential for becoming a human person and deliberately to destroy it.'

Supporters of embryo research point out that women's bodies destroy most potential human beings quite naturally: the majority of embryos fail to implant. The number that die in the laboratory is only a tiny fraction of the number that nature wantonly destroys. Furthermore, if an embryo, as potential human being, is given the same moral status as an actual human being, then the egg and sperm must also be given it, because they too have the potential to become a human being. And yet neither eggs nor sperms have special moral status; menstruation and male masturbation are not seen as murder; and embryos lost during menstruation are not recovered and nurtured. The possibility of human cloning, explored in Chapter 10, reinforces this argument: almost without exception, each cell of your body could be cloned, making a complete new human being, and is therefore a potential person, too. And yet we do not give special moral status to skin cells on the soles of our feet, for example.

The dissenting members of the Warnock Committee were aware of this sort of objection, and countered it: 'neither [egg nor sperm] alone, given the appropriate environment, will [become a person]'.

Similarly with cloning, a skin cell left alone in the correct environment cannot spontaneously become a human being: its DNA must be first transferred to an egg cell. For many people, however, the argument over whether a potential human being should have the same status as an actual person is not the main issue. For them, the important question is: 'When does a potential human being become an actual human being?' The problem is that the question has no clear-cut answer. Certainly, a new-born baby is a person, and people would be horrified if experiments were carried out on babies – particularly if the baby had no chance of survival after the experiment, and was simply discarded, as embryos are. On the other hand, the egg and sperm which created that baby are clearly not a person. This suggests that the embryo or foetus 'becomes' a person at some stage between fertilization and birth.

These issues throw up one of the most important questions of embryo research: 'Up to what point should scientists be permitted to keep an embryo alive outside the body?' The majority of the Warnock Committee recommended – as others had previously done – that: 'No live human embryo. . . may be kept alive, if not transferred to a woman beyond fourteen days after fertilization. . .' It reached this conclusion from a scientific standpoint. Rather than considering when an embryo becomes a person in a philosophical sense, they based their judgement on the embryo's physical development. The fourteenth day is the end of the process of implantation into the lining of the womb, and a few days before the very first nerve cells start to form. It is worth bearing in mind the fact that, at this stage, the embryo exists as a tiny clump of cells still smaller than this full stop. In reality, as the Committee was aware and as was pointed out earlier, this is still rather arbitrary: a fourteen-day-old embryo is no more or less a person than a ten-day- or twenty-day-old embryo. The process of development from fertilized egg to embryo to foetus to newborn child is a continuous one.

It would be another seven years before the Warnock Committee's recommendations were put into practice. The authority proposed by the Committee (the HFEA) began its work in 1991. In the intervening period, a non-statutory body – called the Voluntary Licensing Authority (VLA) – fulfilled some of the roles eventually played by the HFEA. The VLA was set up by the Royal College of Obstetricians and Gynaecology, along with the Medical Research Council. It demonstrated that it is possible to license IVF clinics and to control what those clinics were doing. So it was a kind of ethical watchdog and, although decisions it made could not be enforced by law, it was a useful precursor to the HFEA. It carried on its work through the tumultuous political climate of the following six years. The period between the publication of the Warnock Report, in 1984, and the passage of the Human Fertilization and Embryology Act, in 1990, was an uncertain time for anyone involved with human embryos, whether experimentally or philosophically and whatever their opinion about IVF and embryo research. As we shall see, supporters and opponents of embryo research employed clever political tactics and counter-tactics, aimed at lobbying support for their point of view.

Soon after the publication of the Warnock Report, recalls Jack Scarisbrick, LIFE produced its own report:

'We produced what I think was a pretty powerful response, called "Warnock Dissected". . . Warnock then produced a follow up, which we replied to. The Government, of course, gave its blessing to Warnock. We then organized a petition. It was a petition to Parliament to uphold respect for life from the beginning, and to respect the moral status of the human embryo. We got well over two million signatures on that petition.'

Fighting for embryo rights

Later in 1984, veteran Conservative MP Enoch Powell put forward a Private Member's Bill: a proposal for a new piece of legislation. Powell felt strongly that research could be done in a non-invasive way, without experimenting on human embryos. He thought that experimentation on human embryos would 'open the floodgates' to more and more immoral practices. The bill's title was 'The Unborn Children (Protection) Bill'. As we shall see, the bill was eventually defeated, but if it had been passed – and its recommendations had become law – it would have become illegal in the UK for human embryos to be manipulated at all, except in procedures aimed solely at overcoming infertility. This would have outlawed all human embryo research. Furthermore, couples seeking IVF treatment would have had to gain permission from the Secretary of State before they could proceed. The title of the bill inherently equates the embryo with the unborn child – something that many IVF supporters disagreed with.

Private Member's Bills are entered into a ballot of backbench MPs, and the five most voted-for go on to be considered in Parliament.

Powell's bill gained second place in the ballot, and so went through the necessary parliamentary processes. If Powell's proposals had eventually been taken up, British scientists would have experienced what would probably have been the first ever ban on research. The majority of IVF practitioners did not realize the threat, but a few scientists did become aware of the need to start fighting. One of those scientists was Virginia Bolton, who was part of a small team at Cambridge, investigating the ability of sperms to bring about fertilization. She says her research – which would have been outlawed had Powell's bill been successful – was important to a better understanding of IVF: 'It. . . has had an impact on subsequent research in the field, and on general understanding of human development and the failure of IVF treatment.'

Bolton remembers the moment she realized the effect that Powell's bill would have had on her work: 'This was actually a very dangerous moment, and if we didn't do something now, the future of our research, and research nationwide could be changed for ever.'

Robert Edwards also realized the impact that Powell's recommendations would have. He considered the bill to be 'one of the most serious infringements of individuals' rights ever to be placed before the Mother of Parliaments'.

Enoch Powell's bill got as far as the third reading before being defeated. All bills put before Parliament go through 'readings', votes and other stages – including debates in the House of Lords – before they can obtain Royal Assent, thereby becoming become law. During the passage of Powell's bill through this parliamentary process, SPUC and other anti-research organizations spearheaded powerful lobbies, and this increased support for the bill. The first reading of a bill merely introduces the bill to Parliament, but at the second reading MPs have their first opportunity to debate and vote upon the bill's recommendations. Powell achieved an impressive majority of four-to-one in the vote at the second reading. But there was a long way to go. After its second reading, a bill goes to a committee stage, in which a parliamentary committee debates each of its clauses. The committee stage of Powell's bill saw fierce debates between those who were pro-life and those who were pro-research. Some of those opposed to Powell's bill – in favour of embryo research – used time-wasting tactics to delay the bill, and so tried to sabotage it. Several scientists, including Virginia Bolton, were spurred into action, gathering any reference material that they thought could be seen as remotely relevant to the debates, and feeding it to MPs outside the

Committee Room. Peter Thurnham MP remembers his role during one sitting of the committee:

'I was given a copy of the Hammersmith Hospital laboratory procedure notes for getting the test tubes clean, and I thought that this was something that the committee should be aware of [!], so we had an all-night sitting once and it took me about three hours to get through all of that. Enoch Powell sat there through it all: quite extraordinary for a man of his age. . . close on seventy. . . It was the Civil Servants who had difficulty in staying awake.'

At the end of the committee stage, the committee's chairperson reports back to the House of Commons, with any suggested amendments. Following this is the report stage, at which time any final amendments may be considered. When Powell's bill was at the report stage, Dafydd Wigley MP thought that the Speaker of the House of Commons was allowing it to progress too quickly. Wigley had two sons who died from an inherited disease that restricted their life spans to just twelve and thirteen years, and so he felt particularly strongly about the issue of embryo research, which could help to prevent this sort of sad situation. In an unprecedented incident, Wigley became so annoyed that he thumped the wing of the Speaker's chair, which broke. That evening, the television news reported the incident, saying that this was the first time that furniture had been destroyed in the House of Commons since World War II. Wigley explained to members of the press that 'there was a loose screw in the chair'. The press thought that Wigley was referring to the Speaker, and Wigley had to apologize the following week. At the third reading of a parliamentary bill, a vote is taken on whether that bill should pass to the House of Lords, where a similar debating procedure would then begin. Powell's bill never made it to the House of Lords. Here is what happened.

According to a little-known rule of the House of Commons, a by-election – caused by the recent death of a serving MP – could be debated in preference to any other business. Labour MP Dennis Skinner shrewdly invoked this rule, forcing a debate on an imminent by-election in the constituency of Brecon and Radnor, in Wales. This debate automatically took precedence over Powell's bill, which ran out of time. Robert Winston was watching the proceedings from the Commons Gallery and relishes the memory:

'Powell sat there grey-faced and furious, and Dennis Skinner gave the most wonderful speech, which I shall never forget. It was hilariously funny because he said, "And now we've come to the moment that everybody's been waiting for. . . this great moral issue that the whole country has been disturbed about." And he went on in this sort of tone, ending off the sentence by saying, "It's whether or not the good people of Radnor will be disenfranchised." It was a great moment.'

David Whittingham was also there: 'The whole morning was taken up with – well it was live theatre really, at its best – and eventually [the Bill] was talked out.'

So, despite some considerable support in its favour, the bill ran out of time, and was lost. Powell had a majority of MPs on his side, and there was nothing to stop a different MP from introducing another, similar bill. Those who had opposed Powell's bill realized that the defeat of the bill was not the end of the matter. They realized that the fight would continue, and that they would have to organize themselves. A key weapon in that fight would be education: if MPs could understand the science behind IVF, they would perhaps see the relevance of embryo research. After the Powell bill had been talked out, the scientists and politicians who were in favour of embryo research formed an organization called Progress. This was begun by members of a cross-party watchdog called the Birth Control Trust, which believed in the right to choose abortion. The Birth Control Trust recognized the relevance of Powell's bill to their concerns: any protection afforded by law to embryos might also, by extension, affect foetuses, and therefore the law on abortion. One of the key figures in Progress from the outset was Peter Thurnham:

'Well, it was very important that we had a body that would fight the issue. The other side had its bodies – the LIFE and SPUC lobbies – and we needed a strong body to bring together the coalition of interests.'

During the period between the defeat of Enoch Powell's bill, in 1984, and the success of the Human Fertilization and Embryology Bill, in 1990, members of Progress campaigned fervently in favour of IVF and embryo research, explaining the benefits that each would bring. They appeared on television and radio, spoke at women's institutes, Rotary clubs; anywhere they felt people needed education on these complex issues. They sent out pamphlets and standard letters to MPs, showed explanatory videos in the Houses of Parliament, and organized mass rallies to lobby support. Thurnham effectively ran the Progress campaign from his flat near Westminster, where he had a wall chart, colour-coded to illustrate the opinion of each of the 650 MPs. Over the next five years, while Progress worked hard to gain the support of more MPs, the colours on Thurnham's chart slowly began to change. One reason why Thurnham was in favour of research being carried out on human embryos was that he had adopted a child with a disabling genetic disorder.

Research was, and is, vital in developing genetic tests that can be carried out on IVF embryos, before they are transferred to a woman's womb. These tests – called PGD (pre-implantation genetic diagnosis) – can help to prevent children with severe disabilities or life-shortening diseases from being born. If the results of a genetic test indicate that a particular embryo has a serious genetic disorder, then that embryo will not be transferred. Women's bodies naturally discard most of such embryos, and indeed most would be rejected if they had been transferred after normal IVF (without PGD). Nevertheless, some do survive, and produce children with severe disabilities. SPUC and other pro-life organizations were against genetic testing of embryos from the start. One of their arguments against genetic testing was the idea that it devalues people living with genetic abnormalities. In selecting only the healthy embryos, PGD is indeed a kind of 'quality control'. Those in favour of genetic testing argue that people living with disabilities should, more than anyone, be in favour of preventing others from having to be born with the same disabilities. This is based on the assumption that no one would actively choose to give birth to a child with disabilities.

The history, procedures and the ethics of genetic testing, and how it relates to IVF, are explained more fully in the next chapter.

Chapter 7

IT'S IN THE GENES

'We could remove single cells at a stage at which an embryo would normally be selected for transfer in a normal IVF cycle. And so there was a window of opportunity now that we'd got the genetic material from this embryo.'

Alan Handyside, pioneer of pre-implantation genetic diagnosis

During the 1980s, while heated debates were taking place in Parliament, both IVF and embryo research continued apace. More and more IVF clinics were opened, and more and more IVF babies were produced as a result. One of the most significant areas of applied embryo research was pre-implantation genetic diagnosis (PGD). As explained briefly in Chapter 6, PGD involves carrying out genetic tests on embryos, to determine whether or not the children that could grow from those embryos would be born with inherited diseases or chromosomal abnormalities. Only if the tests show that the embryo is 'normal' will the embryo be transferred. The test is generally carried out on the DNA from one cell removed from a six- or eight-celled embryo. Since its first successful application in 1989, the technique has been refined and used many times, although it is by no means a routine part of IVF treatment. However, new variations of PGD, and new techniques, have been developed, making the whole process more widely applicable and more 'convenient'. Genetic testing before a pregnancy is established will almost certainly become more common.

PGD was not the first method of prenatal diagnosis. Most people have heard of amniocentesis, which can also detect genetic and chromosomal abnormalities. The main difference between PGD and amniocentesis is that the latter can be used only long after a pregnancy is under way. As noted in Chapter 4, amniocentesis detected no chromosomal abnormalities in Lesley Brown's baby. The test also indicated that the baby was a girl. Amniocentesis has been used since the 1930s, and has diagnosed chromosomal abnormalities in hundreds of thousands of foetuses – in some cases, resulting in terminations of pregnancy. This is the main source of the moral concern that prenatal genetic testing brings with it. We shall explore some of the moral and ethical consequences of PGD later in this chapter.

The embryos involved in PGD are generally produced by IVF, although it is possible to use embryos recovered from a woman's body. In this latter case, embryos are obtained by a procedure called lavage, in which a fluid is pumped into the woman's womb, literally to wash the embryo out before it implants. With embryo collection by lavage, timing is essential: too early, and the embryo will not yet have reached the womb; too late, and it may have already implanted. If the embryo has already implanted then PGD cannot be performed, and there is a risk that a child with genetic or chromosomal abnormalities could be born. So, lavage is at present an unreliable method of embryo collection and, at the time of writing, no pregnancies have yet been established with PGD embryos obtained by lavage. PGD is likely to continue to be carried out mainly in connection with IVF.

PGD is not only carried out on embryos (although, strictly, the word 'pre-implantation' implies use of an embryo). The technique is also carried out on polar bodies, which as we saw in Chapter 1 are like mini eggs, produced when an oocyte divides to produce a mature egg. They contain half a set of chromosomes, just as an egg does. Genetic abnormalities in the egg can be detected by testing the chromosomes of the polar body, which itself plays no active role in reproduction. Of course, this is only used if the potential for genetic disease lies in the female partner's DNA, since men do not produce polar bodies.

Testing times
The idea of PGD has a long history. As early as the mid-1960s – before Robert Edwards had even achieved the fertilization of a human egg outside the body – he was aware of the advantages that genetic diagnosis of embryos could bring. As he says:

'I began to think that it was essential to do genetics. . . but you could do nothing about it in those days. I wanted to identify the genes and. . . transfer a good embryo to avoid the birth of children with inherited defects.'

The desire for PGD remained, albeit on the sidelines, throughout the 1970s. Exciting improvements in the understanding and manipulation of DNA during the 1980s made it technically possible and, by the end of the 1980s, it had become a reality. The technique is still not widely used. In fact, the importance of PGD in the history of assisted reproduction so far lies mainly in the part it played in convincing British MPs of the need for embryo research. As we shall see in Chapter 8, the first successful application of PGD influenced opinions about embryo research, helping to bring about the passage of the Human Fertilization and Embryology Act in 1990.

Of course not everyone was, or is, convinced of the need for PGD, and many are not happy with its moral consequences. PGD involves the direct manipulation of human embryos: this alone is enough to send shivers down the spine of those sensitive to embryo research. Perhaps more importantly, PGD results in the favoured selection of one or two 'normal' embryos over other, 'defective' ones (how the term arises is discussed below). Pro-life organizations saw this selection process as a form of discrimination against individuals with disablement caused by genetic abnormalities. It was compared with eugenics, the aim of which is to improve the hereditary qualities of a species. In humans, eugenics is an attempt to direct our own evolution. The very word 'eugenics' has negative connotations. For example, in Hitler's Nazi Germany, attempts were made to eradicate what were seen as genetically inferior people: in particular Jews and homosexuals. Before we look at PGD in more detail, and explore its suggested link with eugenics, it is necessary to explain a little more about DNA and genes in general, and genetic diseases in particular.

As we saw in Chapter 1, your physical characteristics are determined by your DNA. This chemical resides in the nuclei of most of the cells of your body, and your DNA is different from everyone else's (unless you have an identical sibling). The long stringy molecule of DNA inside your cells exists in sections called chromosomes. Of the forty-six chromosomes in each cell, two are the sex chromosomes, which may be type X or type Y. If you are female, then you have two X chromosomes; if male, you have one X and one Y. The other forty-four chromosomes – which do not determine your sex – are called autosomes, and they exist in twenty-two pairs. One member of each autosome pair comes from the DNA in your biological mother's egg cell, and its corresponding member from the DNA in your biological father's sperm cell. Likewise, one X chromosome was in your mother's egg, while the other sex chromosome – X or Y – was carried by the sperm cell that fertilized that egg.

Along the length of the chromosomes are sections called genes. You can think of genes as computer programs, for they are sets of instructions to build molecules called proteins. The instructions are coded in the form of a sequence of small molecules called bases along the length of the DNA. Some of these proteins help to build your body – your hair is largely made of a protein called keratin, for example. Other proteins, called enzymes, carry out specific tasks inside your body. All genes have specific locations, or loci, on particular chromosomes. Because autosomes come in pairs, there are two copies of each autosomal gene (that is, any gene not on sex chromosomes). For example, on both autosomes number 11 is a gene that contains instructions on how to build a protein called haemoglobin. This protein is found in red blood cells, and is responsible for carrying oxygen around the blood. Most genes have more than one version, or allele. The gene for haemoglobin, for example, has many different alleles. Some alleles produce normal, functioning haemoglobin molecules, and some produce malformed, malfunctioning ones. People who carry two copies of a particular 'defective' allele – one on each member of chromosome pair 11 – develop a serious inherited disease known as sickle cell anaemia. The haemoglobin in the red blood cells of sufferers of this disease buckle and twist together, causing the cells to take on a sickle shape. The malformed haemoglobin molecules cannot transport oxygen effectively. The condition is serious – life-threatening – and this is why abnormal alleles of some genes are referred to as 'defective'. Those who carry only one copy of the defective allele do not normally develop the disease: a normal allele produces normal haemoglobin, and masks the effect of the abnormal allele. People with one of each allele are carriers of the disease, and are at risk of passing the disease on to their children. The defective allele is said to be recessive, while the normal allele is dominant. If the carrier's partner is also a carrier of the recessive allele, there is a one-in-four chance that a baby produced by the couple will inherit two copies of the defective allele, and so be born with the disease. (In each of the other three out of four cases, at least one copy of the dominant allele would be present.)

It was an Austrian monk named Gregor Mendel who first worked out how characteristics are passed from one generation to subsequent ones. He founded the science of genetics, in the 1860s. Mendel painstakingly studied the characteristics of more than 10,000 pea plants which he cultivated and observed. He realized that certain characteristics seemed to dominate over others, just as the various alleles of the haemoglobin gene do. He noticed, for example, that some pea plants are tall, whereas others are much shorter. In this case, 'tallness' is a dominant characteristic, and 'dwarfness' is recessive. Mendel worked out that, where the factors for 'tallness' and 'dwarfness' were both present, the plant would always be tall. And all this before DNA was discovered (in 1869: its role in inheritance was not proven until 1943).

So, what does all this have to do with pre-implantation genetic diagnosis? Using PGD, doctors can analyse the genes of an embryo produced by IVF. If the embryo carries alleles which would result in a genetic disease, such as sickle cell anaemia, it will not be transferred to the female patient. This requires effective ways of recognizing particular sequences of bases along the DNA, as well as knowledge of whether a disease is caused by dominant or recessive alleles. Only embryos that cannot produce a baby with the disease will be transferred. At present, it is only used when one or both members of a couple have a family history of an inherited disease. In the most simple cases, determination of the sex of the embryo is enough to diagnose the presence or absence of a disease.

The diseases tested for in these cases are said to be sex-linked: normally only males suffer from them. The alleles related to a sex-linked disease are found on the X chromosome. A male (XY) has only one X chromosome, and so even if the disease-causing allele is recessive, its effects will be felt, as there is no equivalent, normal, dominant allele to counteract it, given that there is only one X chromosome. This is the basis of many sex-linked diseases. One example is Duchenne's muscular dystrophy: a relatively common sex-linked recessive disease affecting about one in every 3,000 boys. Boys who have this devastating, progressive disease lack muscle tone, finding it difficult to walk by the age of four. The muscles of sufferers degenerate because of a lack of a protein called dystrophin, which would be produced if the normal allele were present. Generally, by about the age of eleven, walking is impossible. Most sufferers die by the age of eighteen. Girls do not suffer from this disease, but carriers transmit the allele for the disease to, on average, half of any sons they bear, and half of any their daughters. Those daughters who inherit the disease allele themselves become carriers.

So genetic diseases may be caused by dominant or recessive 'defective' alleles found on the autosomes, or by 'defective' alleles on the X chromosome (sex-linked diseases). There are many other sex-linked diseases besides Duchenne muscular dystrophy. They include one form of haemophilia, in which the blood lacks a clotting agent, leading to excessive bleeding from even a small cut; and Lesch-Nyhan syndrome, which brings with it some mental disability, aggressive behaviour and a severe lack of coordination. Diseases caused by dominant alleles found on chromosomes other than X or Y – autosomal dominant disorders – include Huntington's chorea, a degenerative disease of the nervous system. Autosomal recessive diseases include cystic fibrosis which affects the lungs, Tay-Sachs disease which causes progressive mental deterioration and results in early death and, as explained, sickle cell anaemia.

Good or bad medicine?
From the above, PGD seems to be an important medical advance, some people do not see it as proper medicine at all. Anti-embryo research campaigner Jack Scarisbrick sees PGD as a worrying development for humanity:

'We're not "treating" in the normal sense of the word, which means trying to cure. We are "treating" by weeding out the people suffering from a disease. And that, of course, is bad medicine. . . Secondly, by [having a] negative response to things like Down syndrome and so on, we're taking away the incentive for genuinely trying to cure them.'

The prevalence of genetic disease has only been fully realized since most infectious diseases have been, to a greater or lesser extent, conquered. Over 3,000 genetic diseases have been identified, and about one in a hundred babies has a disease caused by a single gene defect. More extensive – in number and in degree of alteration to the DNA – than diseases caused by specific alleles are chromosomal abnormalities. For example, there may be too many or too few chromosomes present, or a chromosome may be incomplete. A well-known example is Down syndrome, caused as it is by the presence in an individual's DNA of an extra (that is, a third) chromosome number 21. (For this reason, Down syndrome is also known as trisomy-21.) People with this condition are subject to mental retardation, a high risk of heart disease, and have a much lower than average life expectancy.

Embryos produced inside a woman's body that have chromosomal abnormalities such as Down syndrome mostly do not implant in the lining of the womb, or are rejected by the woman's body after implantation. 'Defective' embryos that actually implant and go to term are still not out of danger: genetic disease or chromosomal abnormality is the cause of at least a third of infant deaths. It is clear why some people think PGD is desirable: thousands of children born every year are doomed to suffer severely from a frustrating and debilitating disease, and probably have a dramatically shortened life span. Those in favour of PGD say these children suffer unnecessarily, because their births could be prevented. This opinion is understandably not shared universally. For some, the idea is an insult to those living with disabilities that are caused by severe genetic disorders: it is not too comforting to know that your birth would have been prevented had the technology been available. This is a very contentious issue. Given the choice, surely no one would actively bring into the world a child with some of the symptoms that we have described. PGD brings that choice, and for supporters of the technique, this is the point. For those who are against PGD, it totally misses the point. Phyllis Bowman of the Society for the Protection of the Unborn Child is one of those people:

> 'I remember one of our members telling me she'd refused to have amniocentesis and when her little girl was born with Down, she was told, "It serves you right." I think that's a real tragedy of our times. And one of our members. . . has actually been told by people: "Well, I'd have had you aborted." You know [she] loves her life. People make the tragic mistake of assessing what they think is the quality of somebody else's life.'

During their political struggle against embryo research during the 1980s, the pro-life campaigners called in a French scientist, Professor Gerome Lejeune, to help put to MPs the case against PGD. Lejeune reinforced the argument that people born with chromosomal abnormalities such as Down syndrome can lead a happy and worthwhile life. He was a powerful weapon, because he had actually been the discoverer of the link between trisomy-21, the chromosomal abnormality, and Down syndrome. Robert Winston sees this as argument as a red herring: for him, the promise of PGD lay more in detecting genetic diseases more than chromosomal abnormalities: 'So everybody focused on Down syndrome. . . but there are many [people] that are actually ill in all sorts of ways with heart defects, and other defects, some who are very, very disturbed.'

As mentioned earlier, PGD was not the first way of detecting genetic or chromosomal abnormalities before birth. And it was not the first of these to attract criticism. Amniocentesis, the best-known alternative, is also a controversial technique, as many prospective parents choose to have their pregnancy terminated if the test uncovers an abnormality. Also, the test itself carries a risk of causing miscarriage. Lejeune had publicly called for the procedure to be stopped. In amniocentesis, an aspirating needle is used to take a small amount of fluid from the amniotic sac, a bag of tissue that surrounds a developing foetus inside the womb. Large numbers of cells from the foetus are present in the amniotic fluid, and these cells contain the foetus's DNA. Relatively simple chromosomal analysis can detect or rule out Down syndrome or other chromosomal abnormalities, as well as determining the sex of the foetus, which is useful in diagnosing sex-linked diseases. Amniocentesis is routinely carried out on older women, whose foetuses are more likely to have chromosomal abnormalities. For example, the incidence of Down syndrome in the foetuses of those over forty is around 1 in 40, compared to about 1 in 1,500 for those in their twenties. Amniocentesis can be used to diagnose over fifty conditions.

There are two other prenatal genetic tests that are well established: chorionic villus sampling and alpha-fetoprotein screening. Chorionic villus sampling is carried out earlier than amniocentesis – around the twelfth week after conception – and involves taking cells from the chorionic villi: finger-like protrusions of the tissue that surrounds a developing embryo, which goes on to become the placenta. Alpha-fetoprotein screening is less intrusive: it involves measurement of a protein, produced by the foetus's liver, in the pregnant woman's blood around the seventeenth or eighteenth week after conception. High levels of alpha-fetoprotein indicate so-called neural tube defects, such as spina bifida. This test is normally backed-up by amniocentesis, as its results alone can sometimes be ambiguous.

The ultimate in eugenics?
On the face of it, the advantages of prenatal genetic testing, in whatever form, might seem to be indisputable. But we have already seen that there are those who object to it in principle.

Some people find PGD less troubling ethically than amniocentesis: the former is carried out two days after fertilization, the latter when the foetus is fifteen or sixteen weeks old. Faced with the discovery of serious genetic defects, most people would rather 'abort' a tiny pre-implantation embryo in a glass dish than abort a fairly well-developed foetus from its prospective mother's womb. However, it is just this apparent 'convenience' that disturbs some people, and brings them to label PGD as a form of eugenics. If and when PGD becomes routine, humans will be capable of directing their own evolution, albeit to a limited extent, by the eradication of 'undesirable' characteristics. This idea of genetic self-determination is indeed fundamental to the science of eugenics. It is also at the root of the objection that some have to PGD. As we have seen, many people see the term 'defective' as inappropriate to describe the variation between various alleles of any particular gene. There are many, many traits that are partially or wholly defined by your DNA. Which alleles are favourable? And who is to say which characteristics are desirable and which are not?

Early eugenicists – placing too much emphasis on nature and not enough on nurture – thought that low intelligence, criminal behaviour and slovenliness were simply inherited. There is evidence that some of these traits do have a genetic component, but it is now clear that the environment in which we are brought up plays a much greater role in determining our behaviour than do our genes. There is still much to learn about the link between genes and behaviour, but we do know that the situation is not as simple as if there were alleles for low intelligence or slovenliness. So eradication of this sort of trait from a society (if indeed one wanted to do that) is surely more a task for effective education than genocide or mass sterilization. However, both genocide and mass sterilization were undertaken in the name of eugenics: the horrors of the Nazi concentration camps are well-known, but the mass sterilization programmes of the 1920s and 1930s are not so familiar.

The USA was the first country to pass sterilisation laws, which permitted voluntary or enforced sterilization of certain types of person, including the insane and the mentally disabled. Much of the prevailing opinion was that what was called 'feeblemindedness' was inherited, and led to criminal behaviour. Furthermore, flawed statistical studies seemed to suggest that certain races of people are inferior to others. Forced sterilization is certainly an extreme measure; and, when its scientific basis is at least questionable – as with the idea that slovenliness is an inherited condition – it is clearly unnecessary and unethical. Nevertheless, Denmark, Sweden, Switzerland, Germany and Norway passed eugenic sterilization laws during the 1930s.

Enforced sterilization is not just a thing of the past. Since June 1995, China has had in place a eugenics law. Under this legislation, couples are screened for genetic diseases, and where 'inappropriate' genes are discovered marriages are sanctioned only if partners agree to sterilization. In other countries, genetic counselling is growing in popularity and extent, and can be seen as a type of eugenics. Genetic counselling is offered to couples at risk of passing on genetic diseases. Such couples may be advised to adopt a child, or at least to undergo amniocentesis or other prenatal testing to determine whether or not they may want to terminate a pregnancy. Genetic counselling, in conjunction with widespread genetic screening, really could make a difference. For example, one in about twenty-five of the population of Britain carries a defective allele that causes cystic fibrosis. Screening, together with genetic counselling and perhaps PGD, could eradicate cystic fibrosis in just a few generations: by ridding the collection of all human DNA (the so-called gene pool) of the defective allele. In its aim, this is no different than the extensive vaccination programmes that wiped out the smallpox virus. But the fundamental difference is that this eradication of cystic fibrosis would permanently affect the human gene pool, not just bring a virus to extinction.

So, is PGD eugenics? And if so, does that make it wrong? As one of the aims of the technique is to avoid the passage of undesirable characteristics from one generation to another, thereby affecting human evolution, PGD can indeed be seen as a form of eugenics. However, there are also reasons why PGD is not like eugenics. At present at least, PGD is based on the needs or desires of individual couples, and not society as a whole. Furthermore, for the foreseeable future at least, it is not likely to have any significant effect whatsoever on the evolution of the human race as a whole, or even a particular nation or people.

The question of whether PGD is right or wrong is more difficult to answer. There are two main arguments for the idea that PGD is wrong: one concerns the individual, and the other concerns society as a whole. An embryo that is rejected because of PGD is an individual – or at least a potential individual – that is denied life simply because it carries an undesirable gene. So, for some, PGD is the ultimate infringement of personal liberty. We have already seen that on the level of society at large, PGD could, in principle at least, and in the long term, have a permanent effect on the human gene pool. Some see this as tampering with something that we do not really understand. Perhaps there are good reasons for the existence of what we think of as 'defective' genes, and so it would be a grave mistake to interfere with the natural course of evolution. Maybe it is simply wrong to meddle so directly with something so close to the essence of our being: perhaps we should stop trying to play God?

There are also arguments that convince one that there is nothing but good to be done by PGD. We have already seen that PGD can allow individual couples to avoid the difficult decision of whether to terminate a pregnancy, by diagnosing genetic diseases before the pregnancy is even established. On the level of society, there is what some people see as a cynical argument in favour of PGD. At present, PGD is very expensive, but in the future, it could be routine and relatively cheap. In societies with any form of state provision for health care, a baby born with severe disablement can swallow up health care resources that could be directed elsewhere. So, as well as avoiding the psychological stresses involved – for the parents, their children and doctors – PGD could have wider positive implications for other users of health care services. Again, this is understandably an extremely controversial point of view. Not only does it seem to devalue those living with genetic disorders, it begs the question of what sort of patient actually is deserving of medical resources.

Whether PGD is right or wrong, it is still a technique that is limited in its availability. As well as being expensive, PGD is only available at a few centres, and it promises to diagnose only a relatively small (but growing) list of genetic diseases. At the time of writing, fewer than 200 babies have been produced using PGD: the technique is currently reserved for couples who have a high risk of passing on specific genetic diseases or chromosomal abnormalities.

Plastic embryos
Despite the fact that PGD involves the removal of one or two cells from an embryo – a significant portion of its mass – the embryo does recover from the process. This phenomenon was demonstrated by studies in animals. During the early 1970s embryologist Martin Johnson assessed the 'plasticity' of mouse embryos. In his studies, normal mice developed from biopsied embryos, or even embryos whose cells he had totally rearranged. Embryonic cells develop into any type of cell, depending on their position in the early embryo. Rearranging the embryonic mouse cells at an early stage therefore had no effect on the shape of the foetus or the newborn mouse. While the same is probably true in humans, the most rearrangement

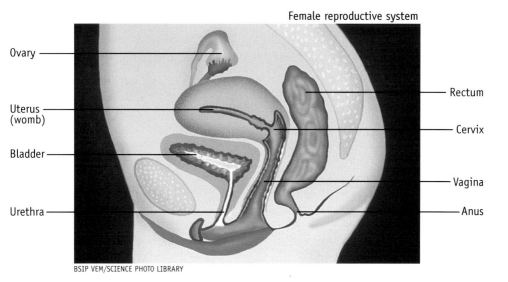

Female reproductive system

Ovary

Uterus (womb)

Bladder

Urethra

Rectum

Cervix

Vagina

Anus

BSIP VEM/SCIENCE PHOTO LIBRARY

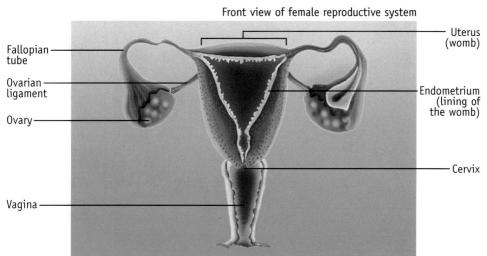

Front view of female reproductive system

Fallopian tube

Ovarian ligament

Ovary

Vagina

Uterus (womb)

Endometrium (lining of the womb)

Cervix

BSIP VEM/SCIENCE PHOTO LIBRARY

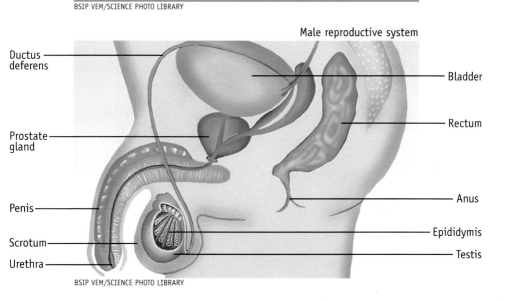

Male reproductive system

Ductus deferens

Prostate gland

Penis

Scrotum

Urethra

Bladder

Rectum

Anus

Epididymis

Testis

BSIP VEM/SCIENCE PHOTO LIBRARY

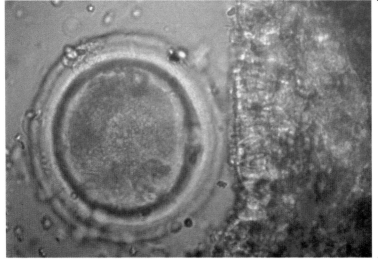

EGG
0.16mm

(1)

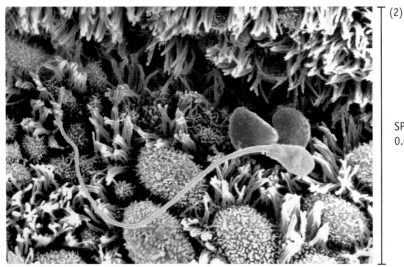

SPERM
0.03mm

(2)

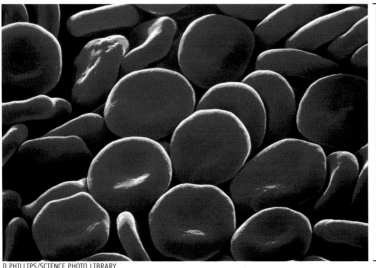

BLOOD CELLS
0.04mm

(3)

(4)

NERVE CELLS
0.02mm

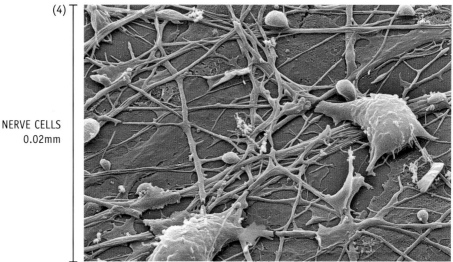

(5)

MUSCLE CELLS
0.02mm

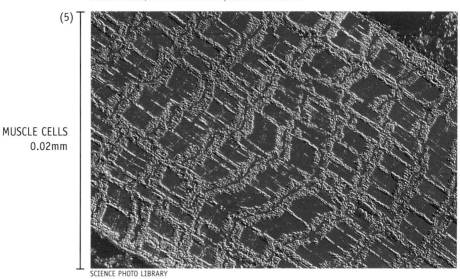

HUMAN CELLS

Photographs of various human cells (see Chapter 1).
The egg (1) is by far the largest, with a diameter of about
0.1mm. The other cells shown are a sperm (2), red blood
cells (3), nerve cells in the brain (4) and muscle cells (5).

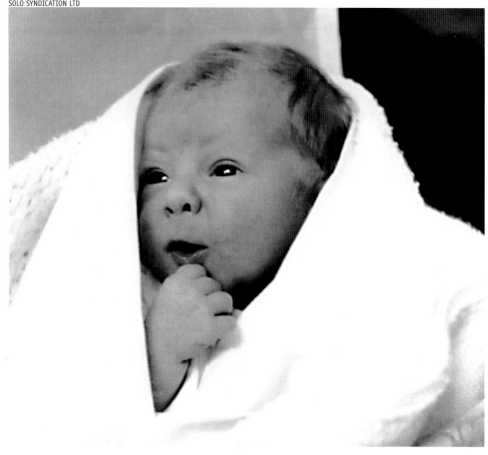

NEW-BORN MIRACLE
The first ever 'test-tube' baby, Louise
Brown (see Chapter 4), born on
25 July 1978. The egg and sperm
that produced her were united
outside her mother's body.

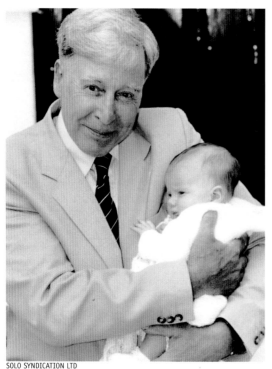

IVF PIONEER
Professor Robert Edwards, one of the
pioneers of *in vitro* fertilization (IVF).
Here he is shown with the 2,500th
baby produced with the help of IVF,
whose first name, Robert, was chosen
in Professor Edwards' honour.

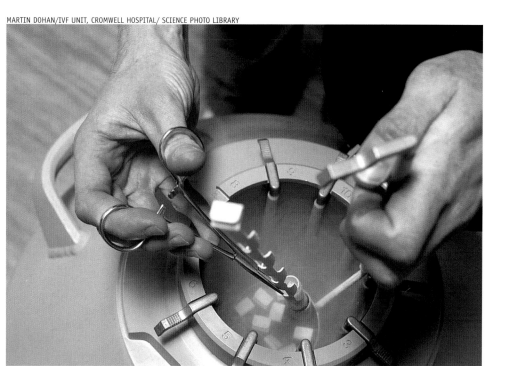

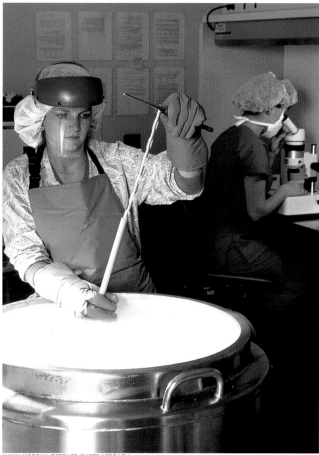

OUT OF THE DEEP FREEZE
Sperm is kept in storage at
-196°C, in large flasks of
liquid nitrogen. Each sample
is held separately in a small
container called a phial.
Prior to fertilization, the
sperm is thawed to room
temperature. Embryos can be
frozen, or 'cryopreserved',
in this way too.

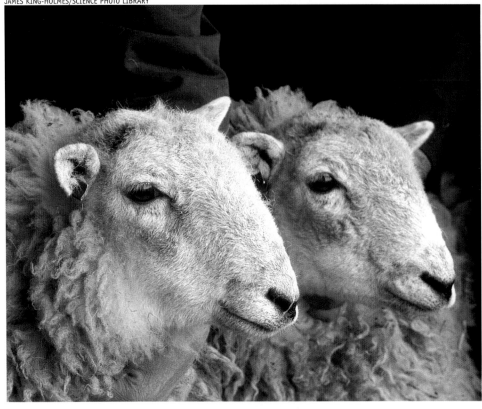

TWO OF A KIND
The world's first ever sheep clones, Morag and Megan, born in 1995 at the Roslin Insitute, Edinburgh, Scotland. The world's most famous clone, Dolly, was also born at the Roslin Institute, in 1996 (see Chapter 11).

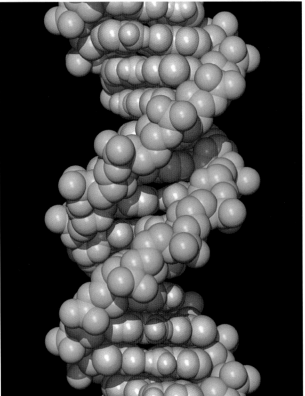

THE CODE OF LIFE
Computer generated image of a molecule of DNA (deoxyribonucleic acid). The physical characteristics of a living thing are determined by its DNA. The information carried by DNA is encoded in chemical units called bases (see Chapter 12), here shown in pink.

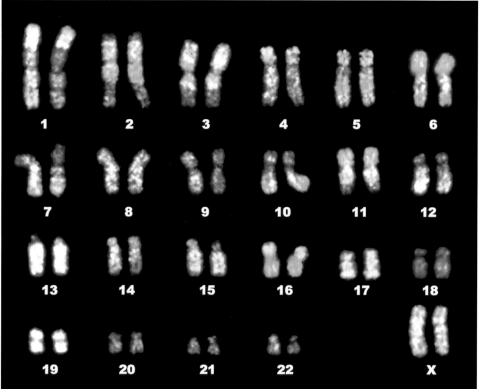

HUMAN CHROMOSOMES

The complete collection of chromosomes from one cell, arranged in a particular order, is called a karyotype. The normal human karyotype has 46 chromosomes: 22 pairs of 'autosomal' chromosomes, and two sex chromosomes, which may be 'X' or 'Y'. A female (*above*) has two X chromosomes, while a male (*right*) has one X and one Y.

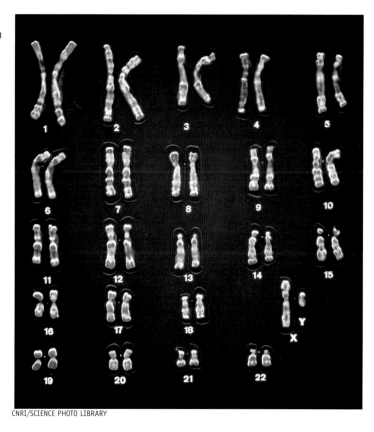

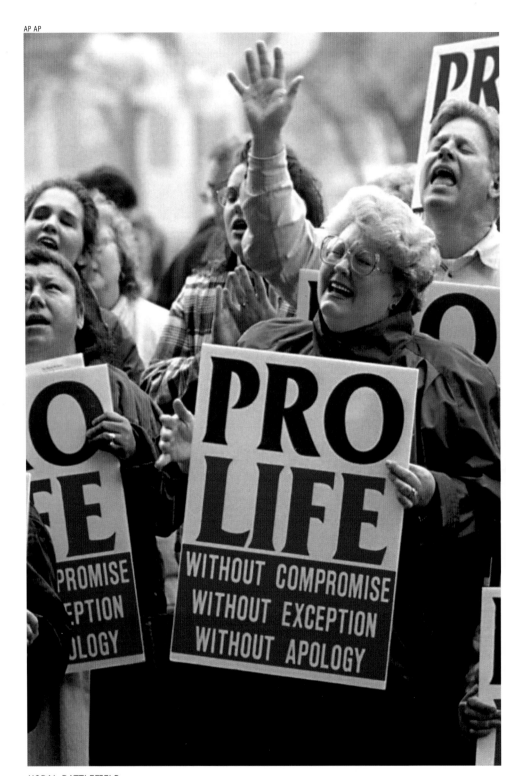

MORAL BATTLEFIELD
Pro-life supporters voice their objections to abortion, on the 23rd anniversary of the
most famous abortion court case, Wade vs Roe. Abortion has close ties to embryo
research, which is part of most assisted reproductive technologies. The issues of embryo
research and abortion sometimes become confused (see Chapter 8).

human embryos are likely to face (hopefully) is the removal of one or two cells during biopsy for PGD.

How is a single cell removed from a tiny embryo? The embryo is held against the tip of a 'holding pipette', and a tiny glass needle is used to cut a small slit through the outer layer of the embryo – the zona pellucida. Then a cell is removed by suction on to the tip of another pipette. The whole process of embryo biopsy takes place under a microscope, using 'micromanipulators'. Movements of the operator's hands are 'geared down', so that a one-centimetre movement of a hand moves a needle or pipettes a fraction of a millimetre. There is a variety of genetic tests. Some involve DNA probes: small sections of DNA that bind to specific sequences of bases along the length of the DNA under test. In one version of this, the probes carry a fluorescent dye that emits characteristic light when ultraviolet radiation shines on it under a fluorescent microscope. Called fluorescent in situ hybridization (FISH), it is a recent development that has made PGD simpler. Another modern invention, which may revolutionize PGD, is the DNA chip: a crossover between genetics and microelectronics. It is like a computerized biochemical laboratory: a square array, typically one or two centimetres square, that carries specific fragments of DNA. Particular alleles, if present in the test DNA, will bind to these fragments. As with FISH, fluorescent dyes are normally tacked on to the DNA fragments, and they are activated when a piece of the test DNA binds. A computer produces and analyses an image of the pattern of fluorescence observed on the chip, and produces an assessment of the sample DNA, quickly and accurately. One array has the capability to test for up to 400,000 different DNA sequences: enough for four alleles for each of the 100,000 or so genes on the human genome. We do not yet know the sequences for all the genes of human DNA, but when we do, chips like this could be used to test for any specific alleles in a matter of minutes.

Developing the technique
The basic procedure for PGD was developed by Richard Gardener, David Whittingham and Alan Handyside, during the 1980s. Gardener, working with Robert Edwards, carried out biopsies of rabbits' embryos, from which he could predict the sex of baby rabbits born from those embryos. In Edinburgh, Handyside genetically engineered mice to test specific theories about human genetics. The 'transgenic' mice acted as an experimental model of how PGD could

be used to test for a genetic disorder called Lesch-Nyhan syndrome. In the mid-1980s, Handyside moved to Hammersmith Hospital, to work with Robert Winston. It was around this time that an important new technique was being developed. It is called polymerase chain reaction (PCR). Although it is not necessary in simple embryo sex determination, for which FISH alone is sufficient, PCR is an important part of the hunt for defective alleles or missing genes. Without PCR, pre-implantation genetic diagnosis would not have become possible. PCR 'amplifies' – produces many copies of – DNA molecules from the single cell obtained by embryo biopsy. This produces sufficient DNA on which to carry out genetic tests. Handyside explains that the technique enables him to:

> 'multiply the copies of a specific fragment of [DNA], so that in fact you end up with billions of copies of this specific fragment. You can then. . . analyse the genetic composition of that fragment. Single cells of course really only have two copies, generally speaking, of a gene: one inherited from the father and one from the mother. It's not possible really to make a diagnosis with only two copies.'

In 1983 American molecular biologist Kary Mullis, working at the time for American biotechnology giant, the Cetus Corporation, came up with the idea of PCR, while cruising along a Californian freeway. He has said that he does his best thinking when he is driving and, for this particular bit of inspiration, he received a Nobel Prize for Chemistry, in 1993. Cetus paid Kary Mullis a $10,000 bonus for his invention and later sold the patent for PCR to a pharmaceutical company for $300 million. PCR is used not only to diagnose genetic diseases. Still in the field of medicine, it is used to detect bacteria or viruses (including the AIDS virus). It is also an important weapon in the fight against criminals: PCR can amplify the DNA from a single cell left at the scene of a crime, enabling the forensics experts to carry out 'DNA fingerprinting'. It has even been used to help research in evolution: PCR has amplified DNA from extinct animals and an Egyptian mummy, giving evolutionary biologists the chance to study this scarce but valuable genetic resource extensively.

The process makes use of DNA's natural ability to replicate. Inside a dividing cell, a type of enzyme called a polymerase replicates the DNA, so that there will be one copy for each of the two cells. During PCR, this takes place in a small test tube. To do its job, the polymerase needs the ingredients – the DNA bases – and a piece of 'primer DNA', which is necessary to start the replication process. The reaction has three steps. Firstly, the double-stranded DNA is 'denatured', which means unzipped into two separate single strands. This takes place at 95 degrees Celsius. Next, the primer attaches to the ends of the DNA strands – at 55 degrees Celsius. The temperature is increased to 75 degrees Celsius, and the polymerase replicates the DNA, by attaching new bases on to the single strands, making each single strand double. So, the result is two copies of the piece of DNA from one. Each time the cycle repeats, the number of copies of the DNA doubles. Within about three hours of automated PCR, this doubling of the DNA has produced over a million copies.

Alan Handyside, who had studied for his PhD under Robert Edwards at Cambridge, was excited by the new possibilities opened up by PCR. Other teams around the world also realized the potential of PCR in making PGD work, and the race was on. In 1987, Handyside started working at Hammersmith Hospital, with Robert Winston. In a frenetic two-year period, helped by teams at St Mary's Hospital Medical School in London and the Clinical Sciences Centre at Northwick Park in Middlesex, Handyside overcame the technical obstacles that lay before him. First, he had to be sure that biopsy of a human embryo would not damage or destroy that embryo. IVF doctors had reported that the human embryo was as resilient as the embryos of other mammals, such as the mouse or the rabbit: human embryos that had been accidentally damaged still managed to implant and develop normally. Handyside used micromanipulators with donated human embryos, to confirm this. He remembers that there was intense media interest in human embryo research at the time, stimulated by the debates in Parliament:

'We had about one film crew per week coming through the lab. There was a lot of media involvement. We gave a lot of interviews and we really just spent a lot of time trying to talk to reporters and indeed the public. We got more interest from patients the more publicity there was.'

Automatic PCR machines did not exist at the time that Handyside was working on the problem of PGD. He remembers 'shuttling the genetic material in tubes between different temperatures' and 'standing over steaming water baths for really quite a long time'. There were many difficulties to overcome in developing this technically complex technique. For example, Handyside had to avoid contaminating the sample: even a skin cell falling off his face into the reaction tubes could lead to false results. The polymerase enzyme used in the PCR – to construct the duplicate DNA strand – was taken from a bacterium, different batches of which behaved in different ways. So, a reaction that worked one day would not work the next. Despite the difficulties, Handyside was eventually convinced that the technique was ready to be tested on patients. A number of couples approached the team at Hammersmith, asking whether the work being carried out might benefit them. They included Mrs Edwards and Mrs Munday: the first patients in the world to be treated successfully using PGD. We shall hear the story of these patients in the next chapter, and how they were involved in a dramatic press conference that swayed the vote on the Human Fertilization and Embryology Bill, in 1990.

Future diagnosis
Although PGD is now a reality, it is still in its infancy. So far, its use has been limited to preventing the births of children *certain* to develop genetic diseases. However, there are many diseases which are only partly determined by your genes. The presence or absence of particular alleles can increase the chance of having one of these diseases. For example, some women are born with a genetic pre-disposition to breast cancer. This does not mean that these women will definitely develop the disease: they are just more likely to do so than those born without the same genetic predisposition. Given the choice of two viable embryos – one of which has a predisposition to breast cancer and one which does not – which would you choose? Since there is a genetic component to the causes of breast cancer, should the predisposition to breast cancer be routinely screened for using PGD on IVF embryos?

A similar grey area concerns diseases with delayed onset, such as Huntingdon's chorea. People with this genetic disease experience very unpleasant muscle spasms associated with a degeneration of their brain cells. Their condition worsens, and dementia rapidly sets in. The disease does not normally manifest itself until a person's forties, and quality of life beforehand is unaffected. Is it right to screen embryos for Huntingdon's chorea?

As well as ethical concerns regarding specific diseases, there are worries about genetic testing in general. Some insurance companies in the USA already ask those applying for health insurance whether they have undergone genetic testing. Perhaps more of an infringement on individual liberty would be a national database of genetic identities, in the form of DNA fingerprints. This would benefit the police, who already use DNA fingerprints to help them solve crimes: access to the DNA fingerprints of a whole nation would help them to identify their suspects more quickly and easily. However, the idea of such a database throws up important concerns. Presumably, a person's genetic profile would be added to the database at birth. With DNA chips, it may soon be very quick and straightforward to carry out a genetic test on a newborn baby, while its DNA fingerprint is being put together. And this would make it possible carry out a 'genetic health-check' of every child at birth. Knowledge of a pre-disposition to a disease could help an individual to prevent the onset of the disease. But at what age should the person be informed of their likelihood to develop genetic diseases, if at all? What other tantalizing or horrifying possibilities might PGD lead to? Could the combination of PGD with genetic engineering be used to produce 'designer babies', for example? Some of the longer-term implications of PGD are explored in the final chapter of this book.

Chapter 8

POLITICAL UNREST

'The credit really does go to Kenneth Clarke as the minister because he put his head above the parapet, decided that the Government would grasp the issue and would go through with it. And by that time of course we had a large number of MPs who wanted to see the legislation succeed.'

Peter Thurnham MP

The pre-implantation test developed by Handyside and Winston was to play an important part in the passing of the 1990 Human Fertility and Embryology Act. Throughout the 1980s in the UK, the need had grown for some kind of legislation over IVF and human embryo research. More and more IVF children were being born, at more and more clinics, and embryos were being used in experiments at several centres. Actually, regulations were already in place, as described in Chapter 6: IVF clinics were regulated by the Voluntary Licensing Authority (VLA). (The VLA changed its name in 1985 to the Interim Licensing Authority, but I shall continue to refer to it as the VLA, for the sake of simplicity.) However, the VLA did not have the legal muscle that the HFEA has now, and some IVF doctors defied the voluntary regulations. For example, some doctors ignored the limit on how many embryos may be transferred to a woman's womb at one time. The more embryos implanted, the greater the chance of pregnancy. However, as we saw in Chapter 5, transferring several embryos at once brings with it a risk of a multiple pregnancy. This may pose risks to the health of the prospective mother or babies.

The first recorded set of nontuplets – nine babies – was born in June 1971, when an Australian woman gave birth to five boys and four girls. Two of the boys were stillborn, and the remaining seven infants died within a week. In addition to the health risks, there is the possibility that the prospective parents will be unable financially to cope with more than, say, two babies. The VLA's regulations allowed up to three embryos to be transferred at one time, in view of the risks. Some IVF doctors – who ignored the VLA's regulation on this matter – found themselves having to carry out 'selective pregnancy reduction'. This unpopular technique leads to the death of one or more of the foetuses in a multiple pregnancy, by lethal injection. Pro-life campaigner Jack Scarisbrick feels that the procedure 'seemed to show the sort of utter cynicism of the whole IVF programme: the disregard for and trivialization of human life'. And yet it continued. Selective pregnancy reduction is now rarely used on foetuses produced with the aid of IVF – in Britain at least – since the law permits no more than three embryos to be transferred to a patient at once. In unregulated countries, however, some doctors transfer ten or more embryos in one operation, to increase the success rate of IVF. As noted in Chapter 5, non-IVF treatments using fertility drugs are another source of multiple pregnancies. Therefore these procedures sometimes lead to selective pregnancy reduction.

And so, with only voluntary regulation for IVF clinics and no moratorium on human embryo research, the technology of assisted reproduction was certainly not beating a retreat. To those in favour of IVF and embryo research, the growing numbers of healthy IVF babies being born were proof that assisted reproduction could do nothing but good. It was helping infertile couples to realize their dream to have children of their own. And, they said, IVF would not have come into existence, and its success rate could not improve, without embryo research. So, for these people, an acceptance of IVF carried with it a recognition of the importance of embryo research. Those on the other side of the argument stressed that for every one IVF baby born, perhaps ten or twelve human individuals are destroyed: and this is too high a price to pay. So they remained opposed to IVF.

Nevertheless, new techniques or consequences of assisted reproduction continued to appear. One of these was delayed IVF siblings: a consequence of the freezing of embryos (cryopreservation). In April 1987, for example, Mary Wright gave birth to daughter Elizabeth after IVF treatment at Edwards's and Steptoe's clinic, Bourn Hall. The embryo that became Elizabeth had been frozen and thawed. Elizabeth's sister Amy had grown from an embryo that was created at the same time, but she was born eighteen months before Elizabeth.

Someone else's child

Another technology of assisted reproduction that gained notoriety in the 1980s was surrogacy. In itself, surrogacy is not a new technique: the Bible tells how the husbands of some infertile women had intercourse with their wives' handmaids. The hope was that the maids could bear children for their infertile mistresses. In modern times, the use of artificial insemination has made surrogacy less like adultery or bigamy. Surrogacy spawned controversy during the 1970s, when contracts were set up between childless couples and the surrogate mothers. This kind of surrogacy was, and still is, particularly popular in the USA: large sums of money changed hands. In some cases, the biological mother (that is, the surrogate) would not give up the child she had carried for nine months. The ensuing court cases for breach of contract, and more importantly the custody of the child, hit the headlines throughout the 1980s. The development of IVF opened up new possibilities for surrogacy: women whose ovaries are functioning but have no womb could be helped to have babies that are genetically related to them. The eggs taken from the infertile woman can be fertilized by her partner's sperm, and transferred to the surrogate mother. This clarifies the issue of custody, since the surrogate mother is no longer the genetic mother of the baby. Surrogacy – with or without IVF – does not always involve a contract and a fee.

Sometimes, surrogacy is carried out for altruistic reasons. Normally in these cases, the surrogates are friends or relatives of the infertile couple. In 1987, the first case of IVF 'granny surrogacy' took place, in Johannesburg, South Africa. Patricia Anthony carried, and successfully gave birth to, triplets for her daughter, Karen Ferreira-Jorge. Karen underwent the preliminary stages of IVF treatment, but four of the embryos that resulted were transferred to her mother's womb instead of her own, which had been removed during the birth of her first child. British doctors Simon Fishel and John Webster were involved in this case. These two doctors were also involved in the first case of IVF surrogacy in Europe, which resulted in the birth of twins in 1989.

Both Fishel and Webster had worked with Edwards and Steptoe at the Bourn Hall clinic. Webster had also worked with Edwards and Steptoe at Kershaw's Hospital, where Louise Brown was conceived. His considerable medical expertise was important for the success of the team. Fishel had been at Cambridge with Edwards during the 1970s. Through the 1980s, the names Fishel and Webster were associated with pioneering work in several areas of assisted reproduction. One of these was sub-zonal insemination (SUZI). This involves injection of sperms into the space between the egg's outer surface and its outer coating, the zona pellucida. This clearly increases the chance of fertilization, particularly for men who have a smaller than normal sperm count. IVF originally had been formulated to overcome fertility in women who had blocked or damaged fallopian tubes. Fishel, Webster and the rest of the team at Bourn Hall decided to make an assault on male infertility. They began to investigate low sperm counts caused by a blockage in the epididymis or other tubes through which the sperms should pass. They could collect sperms from testicles using an aspirating needle – but all they could really do at the time was to wash and concentrate the sperm, and hope.

It was during his time at Bourn Hall that Fishel began to think about how microinjection of sperm would be useful in overcoming male infertility. It would make it unnecessary for the sperms to find the egg and burrow through the zona, and this would be particularly useful for men with very low sperm counts (oligozoospermia) or low sperm motility (asthenospermia). Webster remembers the limited efforts that were made to overcome this cause of subfertility:

'There wasn't an awful lot we could do. I know initially we tried intra-uterine insemination of prepared sperm: what we would do is to get the man to produce two or three samples, aggregate these and concentrate the sperm and put this concentrate into the uterus round about the time of ovulation. We were relatively successful when the man had moderate oligozoospermia, but when the condition was severe, the results were disastrous.'

Fishel and Webster moved to the Park Hospital in Nottingham, UK, in 1985, and they decided they would give SUZI a try. They knew that the technique was likely to be controversial: it had never been tried before, and was unlicensed. So Fishel and Webster went to the VLA to request permission to attempt the technique. Fishel remembers the day:

'We gathered together the info and went to the VLA to make a presentation. We walked in and there was a lovely lunch laid out. So we thought, "They're taking this seriously." But the lunch was for another meeting. We ended up sat in a corner with a couple of people . . . and talked for five minutes. They said, "No: we need more research on human eggs." But I wasn't willing to use IVF eggs to experiment on. There weren't enough. And anyway, I just wouldn't.'

The VLA also demanded more experimentation on microinjection using animal eggs and sperms. But Fishel argued that positive results in animals do not necessarily mean that the technique will be successful or safe in humans – and vice versa. Prohibited from carrying out SUZI in Britain, Fishel worked abroad, in Rome. He set up a branch of his laboratory there, in which he could develop SUZI, and spent much of his time on aeroplanes between the UK and Italy. Fishel resented that fact that he had to work abroad to develop this technique.

The world's first SUZI birth, in 1990, was a focus for international media attention. It was televised by the Italian television station RAI Uno. SUZI became a licensed technique in Britain in 1991, and the first SUZI birth in the UK was in September 1992, at the Park Hospital. Another, less controversial, technique developed during the 1980s was gamete intrafallopian transfer (GIFT). It was developed by Doctors Ricardo Asch and Jose Balmaceda in 1984, in San Antonio, Texas. The GIFT procedure involves mixing egg and semen, and quickly transferring the mixture to the woman's fallopian tubes. This is not a variation of IVF, since fertilization takes place (hopefully) inside the woman's body. Indeed, GIFT is not regulated by the HFEA to this day, except when it is carried out using donated eggs or sperm.

A slippery slope

As experiments with embryos continued, and IVF became more widespread, pro-life anti-research campaigners became more determined than ever to stop what they saw as a slide down a slippery slope – towards a society that has no respect for the sanctity of human life. In the USA, embryo research was all but stagnant during the 1980s, as successive Republican governments, which were generally anti-abortion, refused to fund it (it was finally sanctioned in 1994 – but not without a fight – when the Democrats gained power). In the UK, the defeat of Enoch Powell's Unborn Children (Protection) Bill did little to weaken their resolve that embryo research should be outlawed. Both sides of the debate carried out organized lobbying in a battle for public and parliamentary opinion. The pro-life campaign was already well organized around the time of the Warnock Report discussed in Chapter 6. Two pro-life mass rallies, one in 1984 and one in 1986, illustrated a groundswell of opinion in their favour. Powell's bill had not been lost because of majority opinion: it had run out of time. The pro-life side seemed to have the majority of the public and MPs on its side. Their cause was fought in Parliament by the All Party Pro-life Parliamentary Group. This group had close ties with pro-life organizations such as the Society for the Protection of the Unborn Child (SPUC) and LIFE. Nuala Scarisbrick of LIFE recalls:

'I remember very clearly watching the birth of Louise Brown and, I think like everybody, being amazed and also very moved by what seemed to be an extraordinary success story. I think I started to think, "How did this happen? What went before?" and I began to read and to discover the research work that went before. . . that involved the death of hundreds if not more other created human beings.'

LIFE members wrote a number of articles in newspapers and magazines, and appeared on radio and television, putting across the pro-life side of the arguments over IVF and embryo research. The pro-life side employed a variety of lobbying techniques to ensure that their message was heard and understood. MPs received letters and visits from pro-life sympathizers in their constituencies, as well as leaflets and briefings from the pro-life organizations.

The debate over embryo research was not confined to Britain. The impact of the new reproductive technologies was being felt in many other countries, but Britain was the first to consider a blanket legislation. The world was watching. In the USA, a *Sixty Minutes* documentary examined the issues, paying particular attention to the issue of cryopreservation. Phyllis Bowman appeared on the programme, and came across as very tough, as she recalls: 'It made me look heartless. . . on the one hand we rejoiced in this new life, but on the other hand, is this the way that society should go?'

In 1987, pro-life MP David Alton put before Parliament a bill aimed at imposing stricter limits on abortion. Although this was clearly a pro-life bill, it upset some of the pro-life campaigners fighting embryo research. They thought that Alton's bill on abortion would confuse matters in the embryology debate. One of the major proposals of Alton's bill was that it should be illegal to carry out surgical abortions on foetuses more than eighteen weeks old. The law at the time deemed it legal to abort a foetus up to twenty-eight weeks old. This limit originated in the definition of abortion: 'the loss or removal of a foetus before it is viable' (capable of existence independent of its mother's body). A foetus was traditionally considered viable at twenty-eight weeks old. As baby-care technology grew in sophistication, however, it became possible to nurture foetuses as young as twenty-two weeks outside their mothers' bodies, and this was one reason David Alton put forward his abortion bill.

The issue of abortion had long been a major preoccupation of pro-life supporters. They were totally opposed to the 1967 Abortion Act championed by David Steele MP, for example, which legalized abortion for the first time in the UK. The act permitted abortions – up to twenty-eight weeks – if two doctors gave their consent. The doctors had to be 'in the opinion that the continuance of the pregnancy would be. . . a risk to the mother's physical or mental health. . . or a risk that the baby would be seriously handicapped'. Steele's act was a response to the large numbers of dangerous 'back street' abortions or 'do-it-yourself' abortions, which often resulted in women being admitted to hospital casualty departments. Pro-life groups claim that since the Act, the majority of abortions have been performed more for the convenience of pregnant women than to protect their health; and at the expense of human lives. Leading up to the vote on Alton's bill, they poured their time and money into lobbying support. These efforts were in vain: like Powell's bill, Alton's abortion bill failed through lack of parliamentary time. As we shall see, the abortion issue was to feature again in parliament twice more during the last few years of the 1980s.

During the various stages of Alton's bill, genetic-disorder interest groups had become involved in the abortion issue. Some were pro-life: they believed that abortion of a foetus because a prenatal test highlights genetic abnormality is a form of discrimination. Many such groups followed the pro-life line taken in the human embryo debate, too, and took part in mass rallies. Other genetic disorder groups were pro-choice: they thought that a pregnant woman should have the right to choose abortion if her foetus shows signs of chromosomal abnormality or genetic disease. Some diseases could not be detected until the foetus was twenty weeks or more old. If the abortion bill had gone through, women who discover they are carrying a child with a genetic disorder at, say, twenty weeks, would not be able to terminate their pregnancies. So, the genetic disease groups were split over abortion: some pro-choice and others pro-life. Alliances formed between sympathizing groups on both sides of the abortion debate, and these relationships generally lasted throughout the period of lobbying that accompanied the embryology bill.

The pro-research side used the same sorts of techniques as the pro-life side to gain support: they too produced leaflets, encouraged their supporters to visit their MPs, and held mass rallies. Since the defeat of Enoch Powell's bill, the pro-research group Progress had gained strength and support, but they were in need of funds. IVF clinics were reluctant to send money: perhaps they did not realize that a ban on embryo research could have threatened their entire industry. When the white paper was published, financial support for Progress picked up, and Denise Servante joined Progress as its first employee. As campaign officer, she worked hard coordinating the organization's lobbying efforts. She organized a rally of families who had benefited from IVF treatment. These families – including the children – visited Parliament and explained the difference that IVF had made to their lives: a very powerful weapon in the fight for IVF. Inside Parliament, Peter Thurnham MP continued to be active in targeting specific Members of Parliament. He would invite them to lunch or dinner at his flat in Westminster, and speak confidentially with them. He discovered that there were a number of MPs who had had IVF children of their own, or whose grandchildren were conceived that way. Thurnham made them aware of the part that embryo research played in IVF – a role disputed by pro-life groups in their campaign literature. Thurnham made sure he was aware of why MPs held the opinions they did. With that information, he could use particular arguments with particular MPs. Most important to him were the 'waverers', who could see the benefits of IVF, but had moral or religious misgivings about embryo research. Thurnham recalls noting pro-research arguments from within religious communities, to help convince these waverers of the importance of embryo research:

'The Archbishop of York was a strong supporter of research. Gordon Dunstan, the Queen's chaplain had written on the importance of this research. The Church of England Senate [by a narrow majority] came out in favour of research. And we made sure that those Members of Parliament who had doubts from a theological point of view, from an ethical point of view were informed about those arguments.'

There were, of course, many religious arguments against the manipulation of embryos and IVF, too. In 1990 Anglican members of LIFE, backed up by some high-ranking members of the Church of England, asserted that destructive embryo research was something which the 'central tradition of Christian thought, common to all churches, must reject'. As one might imagine, MPs experienced a barrage of differing opinions like these, on each of the various aspects of the bill.

As an extension of their lobbying, and a way of winning public opinion, representatives of both sides appeared frequently on television and radio. Robert Winston – by now chairing Progress – appeared on the popular television chat show *Wogan* with pro-life MP Anne Winterton. Winston recalls: 'I realized that we were beginning to win because the audience shouted her down. [Terry] Wogan had been very nervous about it. He told us afterwards.'

Television programmes like that began to turn the tide. Documentaries were made, too. A BBC *Panorama* programme did much to gain support for the pro-research cause. Its producer, Margaret Jay, became convinced by the pro-research arguments as she worked on the programme. Peter Thurnham was so pleased with the programme that he arranged for it to be shown on a continuous loop in one of the halls of the House of Commons. The efforts of the pro-research side began to win favour.

Fitting the bill

In 1989, Kenneth Clarke MP – Secretary of State for Health at the time – put before Parliament the Human Fertilization and Embryology Bill. The bill was read to the House of Lords first. Clarke thought it would receive a good hearing there, since the peers, who sit in the House of Lords, are free from the constituents' letters that filled the postbags of the MPs in the House of Commons. The bill had its second reading, unopposed, in December 1989, and so passed to the committee stage. Many amendments were suggested, or 'tabled', at this stage: from both the pro-life and pro-research supporters. The readings and debates continued, with further amendments being tabled, in the House of Lords. All the pro-life amendments were voted out. In March 1990, the bill had its third and final reading in the House of Lords, and passed to the House of Commons.

In 1988, when Alton's bill met the same fate as Powell's, the pro-life side had understandably protested. The white paper on fertilization and embryology was debated at around the same time as Alton's bill, and provided a way for the abortion issue to remain alive. The then Prime Minister Margaret Thatcher quelled the protests over parliamentary procedure by agreeing to add to the fertilization and embryology bill a clause on abortion. A separate bill, brought by Lord Houghton, was debated at the end of 1989. As with Alton's bill, the aim of Houghton's was to reform the law on abortion. However, it did not have the same pro-life leanings. For example, it would have made it legal to abort a foetus – in extreme cases – up to birth. Houghton's bill received a favourable passage through the House of Lords, and this gave more urgency to the addition of the pro-life amendment on abortion in the embryology bill. Margaret Thatcher kept her promise, and the clause was added after the second reading of the bill in the House of Commons, in April 1990. Alton and his supporters were pleased with the amendment: it revived the issue of abortion. However, some pro-life campaigners could foresee problems. For rather than increasing the strength and clarity of the pro-life message, the abortion issue could cloud the debate over embryo research. The pro-life campaigners found their resources divided between the two separate causes.

As the question of abortion became linked to the issue of IVF and embryo research, SPUC decided to try a direct, if unorthodox, approach to gaining support. Funds from a donation paid for plastic models of eighteen-week-old foetuses, which SPUC sent to MPs. This was an attempt to remind – or in many cases inform – the MPs about how well developed a foetus is at that age; and to illustrate why they believed it was wrong to permit abortions of foetuses any older than this. The abortion clause was only a tiny part of the embryology bill. Some MPs thought that the anti-abortionists were 'hijacking' the bill. Worse, some MPs' secretaries – who had themselves had abortions – are said to have been horrified when they opened the packages containing the models. Whether this is true or not, there were certainly those who thought the campaign was tasteless, and it seemed to win little favour. On the other hand, it helped to change the opinions of some MPs over the abortion debate. SPUC is adamant that this was an effective attempt at educative lobbying; for some others the whole thing was a ridiculous and unnecessary gimmick. In April 1990, despite a favourable passage of the pro-research embryology bill through the House of Lords, the pro-life side had felt that they still had majority opinion on their side: over embryology and abortion. Later in April, however, when votes were taken on reducing the limit on abortion to eighteen weeks, the pro-life side were defeated. The government brought in amendments that were based on Houghton's bill. The figure of twenty-four weeks was eventually conceded. However, the possibility was left open of abortion up to birth if the foetus suffered extreme malformation.

The pro-life campaigners did not concentrate only on abortion. For example, in December 1989, LIFE began its 'Stop It' campaign. The organization produced detailed briefing documents for MPs, together with suggested pro-life amendments. They organized many petitions, too, but the most ambitious feature of the campaign was the distribution of half a million postcards. The cards carried the words 'Embryo Abuse: Stop It', and many thousands of them were sent on to MPs. Other pro-life groups organized events to raise consciousness about their point of view. In 1990, David Alton held a prayer vigil. The 'CARE for Life' gathering in the Royal Albert Hall was another show of strength.

Trump card

While the embryology bill was going through Parliament, Alan Handyside and Robert Winston were striding ahead with their work on pre-implantation genetic diagnosis (PGD) at Hammersmith Hospital. The invention of the polymerase chain reaction (PCR), along with studies of embryo biopsies in animals, had prepared the ground for a real test. Handyside needed proof that human embryos can recover from the biopsy of one or two cells. The only way to get that proof was to move from theory into practice, and transfer embryos selected by PGD into women. There was no shortage of people interested in taking part in the trial. Handyside remembers:

'We chose three patients to treat, and two of them got pregnant almost immediately and we suddenly thought, "My goodness, this actually is going to work." It was the most stunning moment.'

The two women who fell pregnant were Mrs Edwards and Mrs Munday – the first people ever to carry foetuses that had had cells deliberately removed. Little did they know, when they agreed to be 'human guinea pigs', that they would become public symbols of the importance of embryo research. The success of the PGD programme was to become a well-publicized trump card for the pro-research side of the embryology debate, and these two women would be proof in the form of two delighted human beings.

In the autumn of 1989, Handyside was ready to go ahead. Mrs Munday and Mrs Edwards were carriers of a sex-linked disorder, which only affects males. So, in this case, only the sex of the embryos needed to be determined. Handyside looked for evidence of a Y chromosome in the cell biopsied from each embryo. If a Y was present, the embryo would be a male (XY), and would not be transferred. First, he used PCR to amplify the DNA contained in the cell. When there was enough DNA, he used a standard technique in genetics research to test for the presence or absence of a gene that exists only on the Y chromosome. Once the diagnosis – in the form of a determination of sex – was complete, 'healthy', female embryos were transferred to Mrs Edwards and Mrs Munday. Handyside remembers feeling more than a little apprehensive:

'None of us really knew what was going to happen. Were these embryos going to survive after we transferred them? Were we simply not going to get any pregnancies? If they did develop, were our assumptions based on experiments in mice and other animals going to be correct: that there would be no abnormalities of the foetus or congenital abnormalities. And at the end of the day were we going to get the diagnosis correct?'

Normal offspring had grown from biopsied embryos of sheep, mice, cows, rabbits and monkeys. But what if humans were different? What if the foetuses that resulted from biopsy of an embryo were horribly deformed? The history of assisted reproduction has depended upon pioneering volunteers as much as pioneering scientists. Handyside reflects on the importance of volunteers: 'I think the couples that really were prepared to go with us at that stage were really very brave people and pioneers equally with us in developing this technique.'

So, Mrs Edwards and Mrs Munday became pregnant, and Handyside and Winston waited and watched the pregnancies eagerly.

It was at this time, when PGD began to seem feasible, that it entered into the debate over embryology. PGD promised new benefits of IVF to a whole new category of patients: couples who are not necessarily infertile, but are at risk of passing on genetic diseases. This helped to cement the alliance between pro-choice genetic disorder groups and pro-research campaigners. For here was the potential to ensure that no embryos with genetic diseases would ever get to the stage where abortion was an option. When PGD entered into the debate, Thurnham arranged for those genetic disorder groups on the pro-research side to write to or visit their MPs. Denise Servante organized a mass lobby of Parliament that featured members of these organizations. People filled Westminster Hall to hear speeches from people with genetic diseases. Ruth Bush, who was working with Progress at the time, remembers: 'It was incredibly emotional. . . people were saying, "I don't wish I'd not been born, but I wouldn't wish this on anybody else."'

This sort of argument was very powerful. Public and parliamentary opinion continued to move towards permitting research. In May, certain clauses from the embryology bill were debated in a standing committee. The committee included MPs Dafydd Wigley and Peter Thurnham. Pro-life campaigners complained that the majority of the MPs on the committee were pro-research. Frustrated, they began to feel like they were fighting a losing battle. In June 1990, the bill went for its third reading in the House of Commons. Five days before the final Commons vote on the Bill, the scientific journal Nature published an article written by Winston and Handyside, describing the success so far in their trials of PGD: two healthy pregnancies. They decided to hold a press conference, which attracted huge media attention. Mrs Edwards and Mrs Munday agreed to take part, and were featured on the front page of the *Daily Mail*.

The press conference seemed to seal the fate of the issue. And to make matters worse for the pro-life side, the government issued a two-line whip – a call for all members of a political party to toe the party line. Some pro-life MPs in the Government made sure they were absent for the vote, so that they would not have to vote against their beliefs. But others were persuaded to vote in favour of the bill. So, with public and parliamentary opinion already shifted towards pro-research, and with pressure on members of the government to vote in favour of the bill, the voting was a foregone conclusion. The final Commons vote was taken in June 1990. Christine Lavery, whom Progress invited to join their committee after she organized a rally to campaign against Alton's abortion bill, was there. Lavery had formed her own genetic disorder group when her own young son was dying from a debilitating illness. She recalls: 'You'd feel high when you had a well-argued presentation from an MP in favour of your opinion and you'd sink low when you heard a really emotive speech from somebody who was anti-research.'

The vote in the House of Commons was won by a huge majority:

the votes were 303 in favour of the bill to 65 against. The vote in the House of Lords, in October, was just as decisive. Dafydd Wigley, the pro-research MP, thinks that it was important that the legislation was a long time coming:

> 'The time that we had bought had enabled people, the general public, the media and Members of Parliament to become more aware of the implications of restrictive legislation and they changed their mind.'

The pro-research side had won a convincing victory. IVF and embryo research could go ahead, under the auspices of the new regulatory body, the HFEA. Many saw the bill as a disaster for humanity. In its summer 1990 issue, published after the Commons vote, LIFE's newspaper *Life News* led with 'Disaster in Parliament: The British Parliament had approved the principle of abortion up to birth, has allowed almost unrestricted use of all forms of artificial human reproduction and has given assent to every kind of human embryo abuse. . .' Phyllis Bowman of SPUC remembers:

> 'One of our great supporters was Professor Irwin Chargav. He was an Austrian Jew, and his work was fundamental to Crick and Watson; a great many scientists regard him as greater than Crick and Watson. And he flew to this country to help us at the time of the Enoch Powell bill, at the time of the 1990 bill. And he said to me, "You know, my dear, I've lived through all this before." This was why he had to leave Germany. And he said, "One of the tragedies is that by the time society recognizes what has happened, you and I will be dead and the people who started it will not be there to pick up the account, to pick up the tabs."'

Chapter 9

CONTROLLED EXPERIMENTS

'The HFEA's creation reflected public and professional concern for the potential of human embryo research and infertility treatments, and a widespread desire for statutory regulation in this ethically highly sensitive area.'

From the Human Fertilization and Embryology Authority,
Annual Report 1998

In 1990, the Human Fertilization and Embryology Act gained Royal Assent. The regulatory authority it brought into existence was the first of its kind in the world; the Human Fertilization and Embryology Authority (HFEA) began work on 1 August 1991. Few countries have laws relating specifically to IVF and embryo research. In most countries, IVF clinics rely on the ethical committees of professional medical bodies for regulation; the regulations, where they exist, are normally voluntary, as they were in Britain before 1991, under the Voluntary Licensing Authority. So in nearly every country in which IVF is practised, anyone can set up an assisted reproduction clinic, without being licensed specifically to do so. Although there is no national licensing body quite like the HFEA anywhere in the world, the Australian States of Victoria, South Australia and Western Australia all require that clinics offering various forms of assisted reproductive technologies (ART) be licensed. Canada should soon have its own statutory authority, too: Canadian IVF legislators visited the HFEA in 1998, with a view to setting up an equivalent in their own country.

The HFEA is based in the Liverpool Street area of London, its influence stretching across all of England, Wales, Scotland and Northern Ireland. The authority's main role is to license centres that carry out IVF, donor insemination or human embryo research. In 1998, 114 centres held licences, and there were twenty-three licensed research projects involving human embryos, at eighteen different hospitals and universities. Each licensed centre is subject to a comprehensive general inspection every three years, with other, more specific investigations during the intervening period. The HFEA employs around seventy part-time inspectors, made up of medical professionals, scientists and 'social and ethical inspectors'. The inspectors in this last category include counsellors and social workers. As well as inspectors, the HFEA has twenty-one 'members', who are also involved in the relicensing procedure, as well as determining HFEA policies.

Members have monthly meetings, and sit on various sub-committees that consider specific issues. At least a third, but no more than half, of the members must be experts in the field of ART or embryology. So the majority of the HFEA members – including the chair and deputy chair – are not IVF experts. These 'lay' members come from a variety of backgrounds: there are business people, legal experts and academics, for example. With such an eclectic cast of members, it is hoped that a wide spectrum of views is represented. Among the HFEA's other roles are the formulation of a code of practice, and to keep a register of all donors (of eggs, sperm or embryos) and all children born from ART treatments. New policies are sometimes needed – for example, when a new technique or discovery arises. As many advances in ART have potentially 'ethically sensitive' consequences that go beyond the needs of individual patients, the HFEA canvasses opinion from ART experts, the government, and the public. Chairperson Ruth Deech says: 'The HFEA's policy of public consultation has earned us respect and approval, if not always agreement, in most quarters.'

This policy of consultation seems to be a very sensible one, given the increasing variety of techniques that are available. In 1994, for example, the HFEA sought the public's views on a potential new source of human eggs: ovarian tissue from aborted foetuses or dead bodies. Many thousands of eggs can, in principle, be obtained from a single ovary, and human eggs were in very short supply. The eggs would be used in research or donated to infertile couples. Many people were uneasy about the fact that infertility treatment using foetal eggs would bring into the world children whose mothers had never been born. Indeed, the consultation document was prompted by a proposed amendment to the Human Fertilization and Embryology Act, which demanded a ban on the use of eggs taken from aborted foetuses. The HFEA received about 10,000 responses to the consultation document: and an overwhelming majority was against the use of foetal eggs in infertility treatment. The HFEA went with the majority on that issue but, on the question of research, it went against majority opinion: 58 per cent of respondents came out against the use of foetal eggs, or those obtained from cadavers, in research. The authority felt that much of the opposition was from anti-abortionists, whose cause falls outside the HFEA's remit; and so they sanctioned this source of eggs for research only.

The HFEA runs a tidy and professional ship, but still receives criticism from many quarters. There is an anti-HFEA lobby in Parliament, for example and also in 1994, pro-life MP David Alton put forward a motion in Parliament, demanding urgent reform of the HFEA. Many pro-life sympathizers think that their views are not represented in the membership of the HFEA. Sometimes the Authority also faces opposition from scientists and members of the public. One recurrent – and perhaps inevitable – criticism concerns the HFEA's delay in licensing some new treatments. The HFEA is, not surprisingly, unwilling to license a new treatment until it is convinced that it is safe and effective. One of the HFEA's members, Anne McLaren, puts this across very succinctly: 'We are a statutory authority and therefore we are responsible and cannot license something that we feel may be too risky for the benefits that it will achieve.'

Some argue that experimental treatments are carried out unhindered in other countries – we saw in Chapter 8 how Simon Fishel worked in Rome to perfect the technique of sub-zonal insemination (SUZI), because he was prohibited from doing it in the UK. British patients had to travel to Belgium to take advantage of the technique. The HFEA argues that caution is necessary when treatments like SUZI are in their experimental phase. It is committed to safeguarding the interests of patients, children, doctors and scientists, and society at large, both today and in future generations. Nevertheless, there are medical professionals and patients who claim that someone, somewhere, will attempt new procedures, such as SUZI, which will then be permitted in the UK once they have been seen to be safe. SUZI was licensed at the inception of the HFEA, less than a year after the birth of the first SUZI baby, in Rome, for example.

As a regulatory body, the HFEA is bound to be the voice of caution, in a field of endeavour that could well run away with itself, out of control. It is certainly true that treatment options for infertile couples have grown in number and complexity in recent history. Before the introduction of fertility drugs in the 1960s, for example, infertile couples who wanted children had but four main choices: adoption, surrogacy, tubal surgery, or, if male infertility alone was the cause of the childlessness, artificial insemination of the female partner with donor sperm. Tubal surgery is so called because it involves physically clearing any tubes through which the sperms must travel to meet the egg. In some cases, the fallopian tubes are blocked, and surgery may then involve the removal of cysts, for example. Before the development of the laparoscope (discussed in Chapter 3), surgeons had to open the abdomen to perform any type of tubal surgery on a female patient; and even then the treatment was ineffective in many cases. Laparoscopy – used increasingly since the late 1950s – has made tubal surgery in women less traumatic for the patient, but surgery still is physically demanding and not always effective.

In none of the other pre-1960s options we have mentioned are the children genetically related to both partners. Fertility drugs do not have this drawback, and their introduction offered new hope for both infertile men and infertile women. Some fertility drugs are synthetic versions of sex hormones – made in laboratories rather than taken from people or animals. Work on identifying and isolating the sex hormones began in the 1920s. By the late 1950s, enough was known about the roles of sex hormones to bring about the first reproduction revolution: the introduction of the contraceptive pill – designed to reduce rather than increase the fertility of the women who take it. Soon after the introduction of the pill, sex hormones – and synthetic versions of them – were being used to treat infertility. Most modern fertility drugs, such as clomiphene citrate and bromocriptine, are not hormones. Instead, they encourage, or in some cases inhibit, the production of sex hormones in the body. These preparations are often used as a first line of attack on both male and female fertility. In women, these drugs are normally designed to induce ovulation, while in men they enhance sperm production.

IVF began another reproduction revolution, which extends beyond the original aim of the technique. As previously explained, *in vitro* fertilization was developed to overcome one specific cause of infertility in women: blocked or damaged fallopian tubes. But the development of IVF has generated a greater working knowledge of human reproduction in general. Some of the new reproductive technologies – such as gamete intrafallopian transfer (GIFT) – do not directly involve IVF. But even their creation can be associated with the increasing appeal and availability of fertility treatment that IVF helped to bring about.

Assault on the male

Another important consequence of the development of IVF is the fact that new techniques for treating *male* infertility have arisen. It is estimated that in as many as half of couples unable to conceive, the male partner is infertile (although in some of these, both male and female partners are infertile). The most obvious cause of male infertility is poor sperm production: normally either oligozoospermia, in which insufficient numbers of sperms are produced, or asthenozoospermia, characterized by low sperm motility. Extreme cases of oligozoospermia, in which no sperm at all are present in semen, are referred to as azoospermia. To determine the sperm count and the percentage of sperms that are motile, semen (normally produced by masturbation) is analysed under a microscope. Computers are often used to interpret the images obtained by the microscope, in order to obtain accurate results. If the shortage of sperm in a patient's semen is severe, it does not necessarily mean that few sperm are being produced. Sperms that develop in the epididymis may be prevented from mixing with the seminal fluid by a blockage. A sample of sperms may be analysed even in these cases: an incision in the scrotum reveals the testis, and sperms may be taken directly from the epididymis using a fine needle.

However, low sperm count or low sperm motility are not the only causes of male infertility. There are many other, more subtle, causes, such as a failure to undergo the 'acrosome reaction'. This is the process by which a sperm gains entry to an egg cell: a small protuberance on the sperm, called the acrosome, releases a chemical that breaks down the membranes of both egg and sperm. A tube quickly forms from the fused membranes of the two cells, and much of the sperm cell – including its precious DNA-containing nucleus – passes into the egg. So, in addition to semen analysis, a variety of other tests may be carried out, to determine the sperms' fertilizing capabilities. The *in vitro* acrosome reaction (IVAR) test allows IVF doctors to discover whether sperms in a sample are capable of undergoing the acrosome reaction, and therefore fertilizing an egg. Another popular test carried out to assess the fertilizing capabilities of sperms is the hamster oocyte penetration test, in which human sperm, having undergone an artificially induced acrosome reaction, are placed in a dish with a hamster egg. If a sperm penetrates the hamster egg, then the sperms in the semen sample are assumed capable of fertilizing a human egg. Such is the interest in this test that hamster eggs – with their zonae pellucidae removed – are available commercially. Despite the test's popularity, there is disagreement over its value. A similar procedure using human eggs would of course be more accurate, but ethically debatable; and in any case difficult, given the limited availability of 'spare' human eggs.

So, is there hope for male patients who find that there are very few sperms in their semen or, worse still, none at all? The few sperms that are present in the semen, or trapped in the testes, may be perfectly capable of fertilizing an egg. In these cases, SUZI may be successful. An offshoot of SUZI – with a higher success rate – is intra-cytoplasmic sperm injection (ICSI), in which a single sperm is micro-injected directly into the egg. ICSI was subject to concerns similar to those SUZI, and it was not licensed straight away in the UK. When there are no sperms present in a patient's semen at all, they may sometimes be recovered directly from the testes, by any of a number of methods. The surgical technique described above, called micro-epididymal sperm aspiration (MESA), is perhaps the most common. In patients who have a blockage in the epididymis, the surgeon (a urologist) may decide to clear the tubes at the same time as the operation. The patient may then have a chance to conceive naturally if SUZI or ICSI fails. Some patients need not have their scrotums cut: in a new procedure called percutaneous sperm aspiration (PESA), sperm are collected through a fine needle inserted through the skin. In extreme cases, there is testicular biopsy, in which a small slice of testis is removed. A few sperms may be retrieved from the testicular tissue, and used in ICSI. The ICSI technique, introduced in 1992, is now routinely carried out in many countries. According to an editorial in the medical journal *The Lancet* in May 1998, 'ICSI seems to be steadily becoming the standard method of treatment of infertility by in-vitro fertilization.'

As its name suggests, ICSI involves injection of a sperm into the cytoplasm, the spongy material that surrounds an egg cell's nucleus, and makes up much of its bulk. Cytoplasm contains the organelles – tiny bodies that keep the cell working – along with a complex mixture of nutritious proteins and functional enzymes. It also contains the cytoskeleton – a web of fine protein filaments that holds the cell firm. Placing a sperm directly inside the cytoplasm bypasses several stages of the natural fertilization process. As a sperm travels through the fallopian tubes, for example, it undergoes the final stages of maturation, called capacitation. Because the sperm is injected directly into the egg in ICSI, capacitation does not occur. However, as pointed out in Chapter 3, sperms do not undergo capacitation in conventional IVF either. The failures of early attempts at fertilization outside a woman's body were often attributed to the absence of capacitation. But this idea was proved wrong. Sperms involved in conventional IVF do however carry out the acrosome reaction, since they meet the egg membrane in the normal way. But ICSI sperms, injected directly into the cytoplasm, do not have to go through capacitation or the acrosome reaction. This is one of the reasons why conventional wisdom concluded that the procedure would never bring about fertilization. This wisdom was backed up by experience: during the 1980s, ICSI had been tried on rabbits and cows: with little success, and no offspring (animal ICSI is now practical). In 1988 Susan Lanzendorf at Howard and Georgeanna Jones's IVF clinic in Norfolk, Virginia, reported that her team's best attempts at establishing pregnancies with embryos produced by ICSI had failed. The team had transferred thirty ICSI embryos, but none of them had implanted. A similar trial in Singapore had also failed to produce any pregnancies. In fact, all the experience and wisdom in the world suggested that ICSI was a non-starter.

Perhaps, then, it is no surprise that when it was first achieved, in 1991, it was an accident. It was Gianpiero Palermo, working at the Centre for Reproductive Medicine at the Brussels Free University in Belgium, who had the lucky accident. It was Palermo, too, who decided on the name 'ICSI'. There are many examples of three-letter abbreviations (familiarly called TLAs) in medicine – including of course IVF and PGD. So, Palermo was keen to have a four-letter abbreviation, as Fishel had done with 'SUZI'. Although his English is good, he had assumed, wrongly, that 'intracytoplasmic' was two words.

Palermo had been working on IVF at the University of Bari, in southern Italy, since 1985. In 1990, he moved to Brussels, and worked with a team headed by André van Steirteghem. Palermo was intending to stay for about six months, to learn the techniques of micromanipulation, but he ended up working there for three years. It was to be a fruitful period.

Like many research teams in the late 1980s, van Steirteghem's group were investigating ways of overcoming male infertility. Following the lead of Simon Fishel, they were investigating SUZI. Using eggs and sperms from both mice and humans, they were attempting to find out the best conditions to carry out the technique. One day in 1990, Palermo was carrying out SUZI on a dozen human eggs. His needle slipped, and a single sperm was injected directly into one of the eggs: right inside the cytoplasm. He put a question mark on its label, and assumed that it would not survive. His colleague later told him that that egg was the only one of the twelve that had been fertilized. And it had been transferred, and resulted in a pregnancy. It took Palermo by surprise:

'I remember mentioning to my technician that we should obtain a pregnancy with intracytoplasmic sperm injection. That would help us to prove that this technique works. And he told me that we already had it.'

A few more accidental ICSIs ensued, with further encouraging results. When Palermo was convinced of the efficacy of the technique, he decided he would speak to van Steirteghem, to discuss the possibility of carrying out ICSI on purpose, rather than by accident, and transferring the resulting embryos to female patients' wombs. Van Steirteghem's team had already tried 'ICSI on purpose' with mouse eggs and sperms, but with no success. New reproductive techniques are often tried in mice before humans, as mouse eggs are the most similar to human ones. However, when it comes to ICSI, mouse and human eggs are not so similar. For it turns out that mouse eggs are not as resilient as human eggs: the rough treatment of the mouse egg in the ICSI procedure caused too much damage. Human eggs do survive the entry and exit of the glass needles, and the deposition of a sperm cell (smaller than that of a mouse) inside it. Aware of the apparent importance of the acrosome reaction, Palermo simulated it – by breaking the sperm cell's membrane before injecting the sperm into the egg. It seemed to do the trick. Palermo remembers:

'I took a motile sperm, and I squeezed the flagellum – the tail – of that sperm against the bottom of the petri dish with the needle... So, I demonstrated you need a live sperm and also you need to damage the membrane of the sperm immediately prior to injection. That's another big understanding, another big step of the ICSI technique.'

This procedure of squashing the sperm's tail is now part of the standard ICSI technique. As well as breaking the sperm cell's membrane, it immobilizes the sperm, which decreases the chance that it will damage the egg. Palermo was excited each time he fertilized an egg with ICSI. But at the same time, he was apprehensive: 'When you realize you have in your hands something bigger than you, it excites you beyond belief. But on the other hand it scares you.'

Cautiously and meticulously, then, the team continued with their ICSI trials. When they had produced four pregnancies, resulting in four babies (twins and two singletons; the other pregnancy miscarried), they decided to publish their work. So in July 1992 an article entitled 'Pregnancies after intracytoplasmic injection of a single spermatozoon into an oocyte' appeared in *The Lancet*. The group's claims met with some scepticism from within the scientific and medical communities, members of which still believed that ICSI was not possible. Van Steirteghem remembers:

'In the scientific community, when I or my colleagues presented the first results, not everybody believed that it was going on. I mean we had many visitors in the laboratory from all over the world who wanted to see what was going on here. And it was only when we had the first of the series of workshops here where we had live direct transmission from the laboratory. . . that the attitude in general in the scientific community changed.'

In the UK, the HFEA at first refused to grant licences to clinics wishing to carry out ICSI. But in September 1993, it sent clinics details of how to obtain a licence for ICSI. It is still cautious about this delicate and controversial technique, and therefore attaches simple condition to an ICSI license: that no embryo produced by any other means (such as conventional IVF), may be transferred at the same time as an ICSI embryo. This is so that ICSI babies can be identified, distinct from those conceived by conventional IVF, allowing follow-up studies to be carried out. The concern over ICSI extends well beyond the HFEA: many ask, 'What if ICSI produces abnormal children?' The same fears surrounded IVF in the late 1960s and throughout the 1970s, and yet IVF babies have essentially the same chance of being healthy as babies conceived naturally. So, is the concern over ICSI just history repeating itself?

ICSI is different from conventional IVF: it involves a much more direct intervention in the reproductive process, and a vigorous manipulation of the egg during fertilization. In 1995, a Dutch group wrote to *The Lancet*, reporting a group of ICSI pregnancies that showed worryingly high levels of abnormality. Van Steirteghem's team had already collected data on over 500 ICSI children, and had found no increase in abnormalities. Nevertheless, some people are wary of ICSI. One of their main concerns is the fact that ICSI sperms do not have to fight to penetrate the egg. Many people have long believed that the 'race' to fertilize an egg is won by only the 'fittest' sperms, and that this is an important evolutionary mechanism that ensures the continued survival of the human species. However, with ICSI, even immotile or misshapen sperms can successfully fertilize an egg and lead to normal pregnancies and normal babies. Perhaps ICSI bypasses a kind of natural selection; maybe we could be passing on genetic or chromosomal abnormalities, carried by sperms that would not have been able to fertilize an egg naturally. In particular, if a man happens to be infertile because of a genetic abnormality, then he could well – ironically – pass on that condition to his children.

What's the damage?
Another concern with ICSI is that the disruption of the egg's cytoplasm could lead to damage – physical or biochemical – of the egg's chromosomes. Some think that this could lead to minor chromosomal abnormalities, in turn giving rise to reduced mental development, or slight or major deformity in ICSI children. Not surprisingly, then, several detailed follow-up studies have been carried out on ICSI children. In May 1998, for example, a team at the North Shore Hospital near Sydney, Australia, published their findings from tests on ICSI children. They compared the mental development of one-year-old ICSI children with children produced using conventional IVF, and those conceived normally. There were between eighty and ninety children in each of the three groups. The researchers found that a significantly higher proportion of ICSI children demonstrated mild developmental delays at one year than children in the other two groups. A second study was carried out at the 'birthplace' of human ICSI: the Free University in Brussels. Ironically, the results of this study were published on the same day as the results of the Australian study. The Belgian research involved measurement of mental development in 201 two-year-old ICSI children and 131 children conceived by conventional IVF. They found that children in both groups were typical for their age, and

neither group scored significantly better or worse than the other. A series of comprehensive, long-term studies will be needed to determine the safety or otherwise of ICSI.

Whether or not ICSI comes with a risk of physical abnormality or slowed mental development, it has certainly opened up several new possibilities in reproductive medicine, and increased the success rate of IVF. For example, ICSI – and to a lesser extent, SUZI – can help men who are voluntarily infertile as well as those who did not choose the condition. Men who have had vasectomies no longer have to undergo vasectomy-reversal operations if they wish to have children. Sperms can be removed from their testes by MESA and given more than a little helping hand in fertilizing an egg. Incidentally, ICSI has been used with horses, to produce offspring from castrated thoroughbred stallions. One of the first ICSI foals was produced by a team in Australia led by Carl Wood. The foal was called Art, short for 'assisted reproductive techniques'. ICSI may be of particular use with horses, which have very low success rates with conventional IVG.

So ICSI is the best hope for men who produce sperm, but whose semen contains none of them. For infertility specialist Dr Andrew Spiers, who offers ICSI treatment at his clinic:

'ICSI has made a staggering difference to male infertility treatment; it has just revolutionized it. We have several pregnancies a week using sperm that can only be retrieved by fine needle biopsy of the testicle. We have men who have a zero sperm count, and yet we get babies for them and their wives.'

The technique may even give hope to men who do not produce mature sperms at all. Sperms begin as tiny cells called spermatogonia, and then become spermatocytes (just as immature eggs are called oocytes). The next stage is the spermatid stage: first round spermatids, then elongated ones, with a growing tail. At the end of this stage, the sperms are fully mature. When doctors take a biopsy of testicular tissue from men with no mature sperms, they may find spermatids. And, believe it or not, spermatids have been used, with ICSI, to obtain pregnancies. The world's first baby produced from spermatids was born in February 1996, at the Nuture Clinic based at Nottingham University in the UK. About two years previously, in 1994, Simon Fishel wrote to the HFEA, informing them that he intended to carry out testicular biopsies in the hope of recovering sperms in men with tubal blockages. He was aware of the possibility of finding spermatids, and wondered what the HFEA's policy might be on this matter:

> 'Eventually, they responded by saying, "Well, we hadn't considered that the spermatid was any different from the spermatozoon" as we call it – the fully formed sperm – so I thought that was rather encouraging. I suggested to them that it might be worth considering it. . . that's where we left it, and they had never said to me at any time that there was a problem in using an immature sperm. In fact that comment was quite the contrary.'

So, Fishel carried on with his work, assuming that he could proceed with ICSI using spermatids if and when such a case arose. And it did. In 1995, an organization called Issue put Gavin and Jenny Oxburgh in touch with Fishel. Analysis had shown Gavin to have an extremely low sperm count. The couple had been advised to consider adoption and donor insemination, but they wanted a child of their own. Fishel agreed to carry out a biopsy on Gavin's testicle, to hunt for sperms to use in ICSI. After several hours of searching for sperms, Fishel and his colleagues could only find spermatids. Jenny, having undergone superovulation treatment, had produced thirteen eggs, twelve of which were mature and ready for fertilization. According to Fishel:

> 'We couldn't phone the authority because it was Saturday, and we had to make a decision. We discussed it with the couple, and we bought time. We decided to inject the eggs. In fact, we found nine spermatids that we could use and twelve eggs. . . so I injected the nine eggs with the consent of the couple, and we decided we'd review it on the Monday.'

On the Monday morning, Fishel found that one of the eggs had been fertilized, and had begun to cleave. Fishel and his colleague Simon Thornton telephoned the HFEA to ask what they should do next. The HFEA was less than pleased that Fishel had proceeded with this unlicensed technique but advised him, under the circumstances, to do what he thought best. Spermatid injection had been carried out with mice, but never before with humans. The Oxburghs were aware of the unprecedented nature of this work, but it seemed that there could be no harm in trying. The single embryo was transferred, and Jenny became pregnant. At this stage, Fishel decided to publish his work in *The Lancet* – and this is when he really suffered the wrath of the HFEA. He was called to a hearing, and received a severe telling-off. Spermatid injection is banned at present in the UK; a situation that the Oxburghs – and Fishel – find unreasonable for two main reasons. Firstly, Jenny Oxburgh gave birth to Susan, who is perfectly normal and healthy. Secondly, the use of spermatids in ICSI is permitted in some other countries; couples like the Oxburghs would have to pay large amounts of money to have the treatment abroad, perhaps in a country in which they do not understand the language. So, why should the HFEA retain the ban on spermatid injection?

Even now only a very small number of babies have been born using the technique. This is partly because it is very rare for a man to produce spermatids but no mature sperms, and partly because the technique is so new. The HFEA would argue that their caution is warranted, given their concern for the patients and in particular the children they produce. Anne McLaren puts the HFEA's case, stressing the safeguards for the patients:

'Parliament set up the HFEA in order to make sure that couples, patients, women wanting infertility treatment had the best and safest and most effective treatment and were not subjected to experimental procedures at an early stage. It is a question of risk-benefit; the potential risk to the patient, the potential benefit.'

Fishel and his sympathizers would argue that a clinical trial is needed, to assess the success and safety of the technique. And Fishel has applied for a licence to carry out the technique. However, some scientists see ICSI using spermatids as unnecessary; they claim that if you look hard enough, you will find mature sperms. Whatever is the truth of this, it is likely that this technique will remain on the sidelines anyway, given that it is very rare for men to produce spermatids but no mature sperms.

Favourable reaction
In 1996–7, Fishel was involved in another pioneering development in ART. This time he was pleased by the action taken by the HFEA. He was approached by a South African couple, Ian and Vivian von Memerty. At the age of two, their first child, Valesca, was diagnosed with a rare but devastating genetic disease called Maroteaux-Lamy syndrome; this makes certain organs swell, causing severe dis-ablement, and endangers the sufferer's life. At the time of the

diagnosis, Vivian was pregnant with a second child. The cure for the disease involves a bone marrow transplant from a suitable donor. The couple appeared on South African television, hoping to find a suitable donor. There was a good chance – three-in-four – that the second child would be born free of the disease, and would be a suitable donor for Valesca. However, in the seventh month of pregnancy, it was discovered that the growing foetus also had the disease. He too would have to undergo the treatment. A donor was found for Valesca, and the treatment went ahead. Ian von Memerty explains the treatment that both children would have to undergo to make the transplant work:

'You have to irradiate and chemotherapy the child to the state where they have no immune system of their own. And they have no white blood cells at all. You then put in the donor marrow through a simple blood transfusion, which then takes in the body and starts to grow and so rebuilds an immune system.'

What does all this have to do with ART? The radiotherapy and the chemotherapy involved in this treatment generally leave a patient infertile. So Valesca was probably left infertile by her treatment. In the meantime, the second child, Oscar, was born. Was there anything they could do to preserve his fertility? Fishel had also appeared on South African television:

'[Ian] had raised enough money – just – to undertake the treatment of his children somewhere. . . that could give them the best opportunity of survival and that was a unit in Manchester. And a friend of his had phoned him saying that they'd seen my interview on South African television about trying to preserve the fertility of children, and that he should give me a call, and this was the call which said to me, "My son Oscar is about to undergo chemotherapy from which we believe he will become sterilized. Is there anything you can do?"'

Fishel had been considering the possibility of preserving the fertility of children undergoing radiotherapy or chemotherapy, by removing ovarian or testicular tissue and freezing it for use later in life. And so he told the von Memertys that there was a slim chance that something could be done. For the von Memertys, it was a 'chink of sunlight' in a dark patch of their lives; but Fishel told them they would have to get the approval of the HFEA. At the time, the HFEA told them, the law in the UK stated that written consent was needed from a patient before reproductive tissue could be taken from them and stored. Of course, Oscar was less than a year old, and could not give his consent, certainly not in writing. However, if permission could be granted, and the procedure could go ahead, then Oscar could be left with the option of having children later in life. He may grow up not wanting children, or there may be no way of using the tissue when it is thawed in twenty or thirty years' time, but at least there is a chance of his having the option. The von Memertys decided to seek some publicity for their cause, and Ian telephoned the HFEA one Thursday to warn them. By the Friday evening, the HFEA provided an answer.

> 'The HFEA, the board, sat down, interpreted the law and decided that it didn't apply to prepubertal [children]. In other words we could take tissue from Oscar, freeze it and get his written consent later on.'

And so, a piece of Oscar's reproductive tissue was removed prior to the bone marrow transplant, and is now in a state of cryopreserved suspended animation. Whether or not this whole procedure is viable will not be known until the first baby is born to people whose reproductive tissues have been preserved in this way. At present, it is unlikely that the tissue would be of much use, but in twenty years, after yet more advances in reproductive technology, who knows?

The sort of tantalizing possibility highlighted by the plight of the von Memerty family has caught the attention and imagination of the public, and has provided a testing ground for the kind of regulation practised by the HFEA. The HFEA's decisions were often in the media spotlight during the 1990s. Perhaps the most controversial example is the destruction of thousands of unclaimed embryos in 1996.

Running out of time
The 1990 Human Fertilization and Embryology Act set a time limit on the storage of embryos produced for IVF treatment. This seems to make sense: if the embryos were cryopreserved indefinitely, then the patients who own them would eventually be too old to undergo embryo transfer. At some stage, something would have to be done with the embryos. If one assumes that an embryo is a clump of cells, with no feelings and no 'soul', then it seems perfectly reasonable that at some stage embryos that were produced for infertility treatment

should be used in research, donated to other patients or simply discarded. The 1990 act states that after five years, the owners of frozen embryos should be contacted and asked what should be done with their embryos. And, if the owners wanted their embryos to remain frozen, they would have to be discarded after a maximum of ten years. Reasonable as this may seem (to those who accept the principle of cryopreservation), the issue came to an unavoidable head in July 1996.

The HFEA was to be five years old on 1 August, and so would the embryos created at the same time as the authority. At thirty-three clinics across the UK, embryos were stored with no indication of what their 'parents' wanted done with them. In the lead-up to 1 August, those clinics had been busy contacting the thousands of couples whose embryos they held in storage. By the end of July, more than 600 couples had not responded – many had moved and not notified a change of address, for example. And so, on 1 August, more than 3,000 embryos were thawed and destroyed. The whole incident gained international notoriety: some pro-life organizations and religious communities demanded that, at the very least, the embryos deserved to be treated with respect, and have some kind of funeral, rather than simply being irreverently thrown away. A petition was presented to the UK Parliament by pro-life campaigners, and thousands of women put themselves forward as guardians and prospective mothers to the abandoned embryos. Nevertheless, the destruction of the embryos went ahead, and has ever since continued to do, when clinics have been unable to contact couples whose genetic material is contained within the frozen embryos.

In other countries, this problem has not yet arisen; but for how long should an unregulated clinic retain human embryos? In the absence of legislation over this issue, couples could request that their embryos be retained indefinitely, perhaps to be born in a hundred years (after being transferred to their great-great-granddaughter, for example?).

Perhaps the most highly publicized case in which the HFEA became involved was that of a widow named Diane Blood. In 1997, Blood wanted access to sperms that had been taken from her husband as he lay in a coma, before he died from the bacterial form of meningitis. The matter was referred to the HFEA, but the authority refused permission: Blood's husband, Stephen, had not given his written consent for his sperms to be used. Blood took the matter to the Court of Appeal and, after a long legal battle, she was given permission to export the sperms to Belgium, where she could be inseminated with them. And so, in March 1998, Blood became pregnant by her dead husband, and in December 1998 she gave birth to a healthy baby boy.

To regulate or not to regulate?

So: is it necessary to have a statutory body such as the HFEA presiding over ART? Cases like Diane Blood's are isolated incidents, and the patients involved are likely to fight for what they see as their rights to determine their own reproductive futures. More generally, is it important to have statutory regulation on specific practices? Ethical committees of medical research councils or health authorities provide a source of regulation, and it is hoped that individual doctors and scientists have their own moral sense that will guide their work. From this point of view, and given that each couple seeking treatment is unique, an organization imposing blanket regulation seems unnecessary. Furthermore, many argue that there is no way of stopping new ART techniques from developing. There will be no shortage of patients willing to volunteer, and no shortage of scientists and doctors keen to try out new techniques – whether for financial reward, notoriety, or simply out of curiosity and a desire to help infertile couples to have children of their own.

Those who are in favour of the sort of legislation enacted through the HFEA point to the need for legal muscle in arresting the development of new developments that may result in harm to the patients or the children they produce. The strict licensing of clinics also guards against malpractice: in countries with no statutory regulation, anyone can set up a clinic, and there is much money to be made. This could attract some unscrupulous practitioners. In the USA, the pioneer of the GIFT technique, Ricardo Asch, and his colleagues were investigated for serious fraud, and, perhaps more serious, for donating embryos from one couple to another, without consent. There are also stories of IVF doctors using their own sperm to fertilize eggs, again without consent – another, less ethical, approach to overcoming male infertility. Though the presence of a statutory watchdog such as the HFEA cannot eliminate all bad or unethical practice, the licensing procedure, with its regular investigations, certainly goes some way towards it.

In addition to the policing of ART clinics, the HFEA takes a wider view of the whole emerging ART field. What are the dangers of

ART? We have mentioned the possibility of retarded mental development as a result of ICSI. Long-term studies should bring to light the truth of that issue. Another claim by some people is that the drugs that bring about superovulation can cause ovarian cancer. Certainly, a small proportion of women suffer ill effects from the procedure, but this 'ovarian hyperstimulation syndrome' is well documented, and predictable in many cases. The link to ovarian cancer is by no means confirmed, however. Fertility drugs have been used since the 1960s, and no link has been demonstrated between their use and ovarian cancer. However, there are many women suffering the disease who feel that its onset was caused by the use of the drugs. This may all become academic: there are many researchers who are looking for ways of producing the eggs they need to maintain the success rates of IVF without the use of superovulation. There could be other dangers that we cannot predict, and that will only come to light in generations to come, when it is too late to do anything about them. So caution is necessary, and, as we have seen, organizations like the HFEA can be that voice of caution. Some maintain that caution is an essential part of the scientific approach to advances in medicine.

Those in favour of legislation also point out that it is essential to consider the wider implications of ART: beyond the individual patients and doctors. How is society's attitude to reproduction changing as ART develops? And can we control that? Whether or not more countries adopt legislation like that in the UK, the rate of of caution. Some maintain that caution is an essential part of the scientific approach to advances in medicine.

Those in favour of legislation also point out that it is essential to consider the wider implications of ART: beyond the individual patients and doctors. How is society's attitude to reproduction changing as ART develops? And can we control that? Whether or not more countries adopt legislation like that in the UK, the rate of progress in ART is unlikely to diminish, and the future will certainly see many more choices for people who want to make babies – if they can afford it. In Chapter 10, we shall take a whistle-stop tour of some of these new opportunities.

Chapter 10

NEW HORIZONS

'Every time we have an embryo, we want to have a foetus and a normal baby. That really is the aim of assisted reproductive technology research.'

Jacques Cohen, reproductive biologist

IVF was just the initial stage of a reproduction revolution. The 1980s saw new techniques, with new acronyms, such as PGD, GIFT, SUZI. And the developments in both the science and technologies of human reproduction continued in the 1990s, and have spawned a crop of yet more acronyms: ICSI, MESA and PESA to name but three. Underlying much of this bewildering array of new reproductive opportunities are the same desires that drove Robert Edwards and Patrick Steptoe to pursue IVF in the first place: the deep-seated need that many people feel to have their own healthy children; and the quest for greater and more intimate scientific understanding of our own reproductive origins. The drive towards safer, more reliable infertility treatment continues. But the consequences of IVF are set to go beyond that.

The phrase 'infertility treatment' has given way to 'assisted reproductive technology' (ART), since the techniques involved are no longer only for those who are infertile or in danger of passing on debilitating genetic diseases. Some of the new options will enable people to 'engineer' their own reproductive lives – to enable women to delay the birth of their first child until after they have established their careers, for example. In this chapter, we shall explore some of the ground-breaking advances in ART that may change the lives of both infertile and fertile people.

Those who take a cynical view of the ART industry see it as a way for entrepreneurial capitalists to take advantage of vulnerable 'consumers', with technology that is far from perfect. The success rate of conventional IVF is comparable with the chance of fertilization of an egg in the natural way, although it typically varies between 10 and 30 per cent, depending on the clinic. This means that many couples spend large sums of money for nothing. Quoted in the magazine *New Scientist* in 1992, the then chairman of the HFEA, Colin Campbell, stipulated that clinics offering IVF 'must offer and make available to all patients suitable counselling services'. One of the aims of this counselling – in addition to simply explaining the procedure that patients are undertaking – is to ensure that patients are aware of the risk that they may not get what they want, and to prepare them for that eventuality. Despite the still low success rates of IVF, there is a huge market for reproductive technology, which is unlikely to diminish in the foreseeable future.

Boy or girl
One aspect of ART that is rapidly developing is sex selection: choosing the sex of your child. The desire – or in some cases pressure – to have a child of a particular sex can be so great as to lead to late abortion or even infanticide. Reports from China have claimed the existence of 'dying rooms', in which female babies are left to die. Whether this is true or not, it is certainly true that some cultures show strong preferences for boys. But cultural pressures are not the only reasons for sex selection. We saw in Chapter 7 that pre-implantation genetic diagnosis provides a way to screen a selection of embryos produced by IVF, to analyse their genetic make-up. This can enable the transfer of only those embryos of a particular sex, to help certain couples avoid passing on sex-linked genetic disorders.

There are other methods of sex selection, not all of them involving IVF, and not all of them designed to avoid the birth of babies with genetic diseases. Long ago, before science took hold of reproduction, people relied on some strange methods to ensure that a new baby would be of the chosen sex. The strategies ranged from placing a hammer underneath the bed to tying off a man's left testicle (don't try this at home! It doesn't work, and can be painful). Needless to say, none of these approaches stands up to rigorous testing. In more recent times, a basic understanding of how reproduction works led to many attempts to control it. The acclaimed Billings method, for example, aims to increase or decrease the chances of pregnancy, based on careful observation of the female reproductive organs over the monthly cycle. Its inventors claim that it can be adapted to favour the conception of one sex or the other. In 1984, American IVF pioneer Landrum Shettles co-authored a book, with David Rorvik, called

Choosing the Sex of Your Baby. Various natural methods of achieving sex selection are detailed in the book, the main one being the timing of intercourse as close as possible to ovulation. This is supposed to increase the chance of conceiving a boy. There are several other methods involving carefully planned intercourse – based on the varying chances of conceiving a particular sex at different phases of a woman's monthly cycle. One is even based on the variation of electric charge of the egg and the sperms. None of these methods has been proved to be effective.

The high-tech approaches to sex selection, brought about by the heightened interest in ART, are generally based on the identification of sperms. As described earlier, the sex of an embryo – and the baby into which it can develop – is determined by the sex chromosomes, which may be type 'X' or type 'Y'. The gametes (eggs and sperms) each carry just one sex chromosome. The egg, produced by a woman (XX), always carries an X chromosome; on the other hand, sperms, coming from a man (XY), may carry either an X or a Y. So, the sex of any particular embryo is determined by the sperm that fertilized the egg from which that embryo grows. One approach to sex selection is therefore to separate 'male' sperms (that carry a Y chromosome) from 'female' ones (that carry an X chromosome). Artificial insemination, conventional IVF or ICSI can then be carried out with the selected sperms of one type, to guarantee that fertilization will give rise to an embryo of a particular sex.

During the 1960s, Landrum Shettles carried out extensive investigations on sperms, based on his hypothesis that X-carrying and Y-carrying sperms should appear different from each other. The intention was to make sex selection a reality through the separation of the two different types of sperm. Eventually, he noticed that there were indeed two different types of sperm: one type had small, round heads and the other had larger, more oval heads. He guessed that the smaller ones carried the Y chromosome, and confirmed this idea by studying families with long histories of children of predominantly one sex. Later still, he noticed that Y-bearing sperms are smaller, 'swim' faster but do not survive as long as X-bearing ones. This was the basis of his suggestion that the sex of a child can be determined by the time of the intercourse that conceives it. Intercourse near the time of ovulation, he argued, is likely to give rise to a male child, as the fast, short-lived Y-bearing sperms are more likely to reach the egg first. Intercourse at other times is more likely to lead to a girl, since many of the Y-bearing sperms will have died.

A related technique of sperm separation, developed in the 1970s by American doctor Larry Ericsson, involves placing sperms into egg albumen and making them 'fight' to get through it. Ericsson has made his fortune from the technique, which he has licensed to clinics worldwide. However, the success rate is not as high as couples might hope – and certainly not high enough to guarantee couples carrying sex-linked genetic disorders a healthy baby. Ericsson's technique can increase a couple's chance of bearing a girl from around 50 per cent to between 65 and 70 per cent. A newer technique, introduced in 1998, comes with a far higher degree of success: about 92 per cent in its first reported clinical trial. 'MicroSort' was developed by geneticist Edward Fugger at the Genetics and IVF Centre in Fairfax, Virginia, USA. The high-tech approach taken in MicroSort relies upon the fact that the X chromosome carries a greater amount of DNA than the Y chromosome (about 2.8 per cent more). Fluorescent molecules are made to attach to the DNA, and the sperms passed under ultraviolet light, which causes the molecules to emit light: the more light emitted, the more DNA is present in a particular sperm. This allows an automatic machine – a flow cytometer – to sort large numbers of individual sperms quickly and with a high degree of accuracy. The approach was originally developed for use with animals, by Larry Johnson, at the US Department of Agriculture, in 1987. The difference in DNA content between X- and Y-bearing sperms is greater in animals than it is in humans, and this is one reason why it took so long for the technique to be offered to people. The other, of course, is that scientists wanted to ensure that the procedure is safe. Some scientists expressed concern about the possible ill effects of attaching the fluorescent 'probes' to the DNA, for example. However, more than 400 animals – rabbits, pigs, sheep and cows – had been born as a result of the technique, and there was no sign of any abnormalities being introduced. Fugger published the results of a clinical trial of MicroSort in the *Journal of Reproductive Medicine*. He does not see a problem with the application of the technique for 'social reasons', an approach that is prohibited in several countries:

'Our perspective is that couples should have the ability to choose their families and make reproductive choices in their personal lives, and that's why in this clinical trial we are accepting patients who have children of primarily of one sex and want another child of the opposite sex.'

The possibility that a couple can actaully select the sex of their baby makes some people uneasy. Will this technique lead to a skewing of the natural balance between males and females? Probably not: most of the people who apply to the various sex selection clinics around the world do so to balance the genders of children in their family.

Age concern

Sex selection is not the only area of ART that is bringing people new reproductive choices. New opportunities are opening up for older women who want to conceive and give birth. As we have already mentioned in Chapter 7, the risk of a baby being born with chromosome defects such as Down syndrome or spina bifida increases with the mother's age. This is mainly because the eggs produced by women approaching menopause are more likely to suffer from chromosome defects, caused by imperfections intro-duced during the late stages of oocyte maturation. But even without the added worry of the chance of giving birth to babies with chromosome defects, a woman's fertility naturally decreases with age, eventually disappearing at menopause. The increased likeli-hood of chromosomal abnormality introduced as eggs mature is one reason for this: embryos with chromosomal abnormalities are less likely to implant than those without. Also more likely in older women are hormone imbalances, and physical problems such as fibroids (tumours in the womb) and endometriosis (in which fragments of the lining of the womb embed and grow in the fallopian tubes). Another factor affecting the reproductive success of some older women is the age of their partners. Older heterosexual women are generally more likely to have older men as their partners. Although men continue to produce sperms until an old age, the average 'quality' of sperms generally decreases with age.

An investigation into mouse sperms was carried out by Christi Walter at the University of Texas Health Science Center in 1998. The study points to the existence of a kind of screening mechanism that helps to ensure mistakes in the DNA (mutations) introduced during spermatogenesis are minimised. Sperms produced by older mice are much more likely to carry mutations, suggesting that this screening mechanism breaks down with age. And this is likely to be true in humans too. IVF doctor Ian Craft believes that age should be taken into account when assessing a couple's needs. Writing in 1998 in the magazine *GP*, he puts forward the idea of a 'fertility score' for women, depending on a number of factors, including the woman's age; the number of embryos transferred should depend upon the score, he believes. As yet, the law in the UK remains unchanged: no more than three embryos may be transferred to any patient at one time, irrespective of their age.

What other options are there for women who are approaching menopause? Higher-than-normal doses of fertility drugs is one possibility. Another is 'assisted hatching' – cutting through the zona pellucida that surrounds an early embryo can help it to implant into the lining of the womb. The possibility of using a low-power laser to achieve this has also been investigated. These options do not overcome the problem of increased chromosome abnormality in the eggs produced. At present, the only effective way around this is to use eggs from donors. Of course, the baby that can result from IVF with egg donation will not be related to the woman in this case. A possible way around this is discussed below.

There are those who think it wrong for older women to be helped to have children. Objections range from the social – some people think that older mothers are more likely to be 'out of touch' with the generation in which their children will grow up – to the moral: if nature, or God, had intended older women to have children, then fertility would not diminish with age. Other commentators, however, see nothing morally wrong with older women having children. In fact, a long-term study conducted by Julia Berryman of Leicester University, UK, indicates that older couples produce more articulate and well-balanced children. Whether right or wrong, increasing numbers of older women are seeking fertility treatment. A menopausal IVF patient needs donated eggs. The IVF clinic finds a donor – who remains anonymous – trying to match characteristics with the prospective mother. Eggs are collected from the donor, and are fertilized and transferred to the patient's womb. The hormonal changes that a woman's body experiences through menopause do more than cease ovulation. Another consequence is that the lining of the womb is no longer capable of retaining an embryo. So part of the procedure of enabling menopausal women to give birth is hormone replacement therapy (HRT). A fifty-year-old woman who was treated by Ian Craft at the Wellington Hospital in London, remembers:

'When you start your treatment you're given HRT, which then will stimulate your womb lining to thicken again and to become ready to accept the embryos. I took [hormones] for four months. And at the point when the donor was... going to have her treatment for her to produce the eggs, when my womb was ready, exactly ready, then I had to have another injection which stops you producing any oestrogen whatsoever, and that for me was the worst bit because that made me feel very depressed.'

Despite this unsettling side to the treatment, this particular patient did give birth to a much-wanted son. Although it is not common for menopausal women to give birth, it has certainly become more routine. In 1994, thanks to the pioneering IVF treatments of Italian doctor Severino Antinori, one woman became the oldest ever to give birth, at sixty-two. Antinori's practice is situated close to the Vatican, which denounced his work as 'horrible and grotesque'.

A clinical delay

While some women delay their child-bearing days for social or career reasons, others may want to for medical reasons. As we saw in Chapter 5, chemotherapy and radiotherapy, while increasingly effective in eradicating cancers, can leave women (and men) infertile. Cryopreservation of embryos can enable couples effectively to retain their fertility after chemotherapy or radiotherapy. The embryos can be thawed and transferred long after the cancer has been (hopefully) eradicated. In Chapter 9, we saw how testicular tissue has been preserved with the same hope in mind. But what about ovarian tissue? A tiny piece of an ovary may contain thousands of potential eggs. In 1995, Roger Gosden and his team at the University of Leeds grafted human ovarian tissue into the kidneys of mice that had been genetically engineered to produce hCG hormone (human chorionic gonadotrophin). Normal human eggs matured in the mice, showing that a graft of ovarian tissue, given the right 'hormonal environment', can reinstate itself and produce eggs. In a bizarre version of this experiment, a piece of ovary taken from an African elephant was grafted on to a mouse's ovary. The mouse proceeded to manufacture elephant eggs. The opportunities opened up by these experiments, for women about to undergo cancer treatment, are clear: pieces of their ovarian tissue can be frozen, and then later grafted on to their ovaries. Volunteers, mostly awaiting treatment for cancer, have already had some ovarian tissue removed, laparoscopically, and frozen. A twenty-five-year-old patient who had suffered breast cancer and had a breast removed was about to begin a strenuous nine-month treatment involving chemotherapy and radiotherapy.

She was referred to Dr Adrian Lower, who removed and froze a small piece of one of her ovaries. Why was she prepared to endure through the procedure of laparoscopy, to obtain some of her ovarian tissue, in addition to all the other hospital procedures she was going through?

'It wasn't the most paramount thing in my mind at the time, I must admit. Obviously the cancer takes over everything and that's what you fight. This was given to me because I was young and I didn't know what was ahead of me. In ten years' time I may well want children. It was an option.'

In a patient with a 'localized' cancer not affecting the ovaries, this approach may be effective: some of her tissue can be grafted back on to her ovary long after the cancer treatment, and begin producing eggs once more. However, if the cancer has affected a woman's reproductive tissue, there is a potential problem. This came to light in experiments, again with mice, carried out by Dr Jillian Shaw at Monash University in Melbourne, Australia:

'Our freeze–thaw methods are gentle enough for all cells in the ovary to survive, including cancer cells. So if there were cancer cells in that tissue at the time of collection then when we thaw it out years later it will still contain cancer cells. And then if we put it back in the woman, there is a possibility – it's not guaranteed but there is a possibility – that those cancer cells will become re-established and re-initiate the cancer.'

One way around this is to ensure that the ovarian tissue is taken when the patient is in remission (when the cancer cells have been killed by chemotherapy or radiotherapy). This would ensure that the tissue was cancer-free, preventing the redevelopment of cancer after the graft. However, the cancer treatment that took the patient into remission may already have impaired her fertility, by damaging the immature eggs inside the ovarian tissue. Another possible way around the problem would be to mature the eggs *in vitro* – outside the patient's body – from pre-treatment ovarian tissue that had been removed, frozen and then thawed. All of a woman's oocytes – from which eggs develop – are present before birth, and so cannot be cancerous even if the tissues that surround them are. What if IVF doctors could 'harvest' the eggs from the ovarian tissue, and fertilize them using conventional IVF or ICSI? Could this approach work?

As we have seen, eggs go through various stages of maturation; only once they are mature are they released from the ovary, ready to be fertilized. An ovary may contain hundreds of thousands of eggs at their very earliest stage of development (as primordial oocytes). In the early 1980s, Bob Moor at the Institute of Animal Physiology in Cambridge, UK, managed to produce and fertilize eggs from immature oocytes, but not at this primordial stage. Only about ten such 'resting oocytes' are present in an ovary at any one time. The oocytes Moor used were taken from the ovaries of slaughtered sheep and cows. He fertilized them *in vitro*, and transferred the resulting embryos to live female animals. Normal sheep and cows were born as a result.

In 1996 eggs were actually matured from their very earliest, primordial, stage. John Eppig and Marilyn O'Brien at the Jackson Laboratory in Maine, USA, grew fully mature eggs from primordial oocytes taken from mouse ovaries. The ovaries were left in a culture medium for eight days, after which an enzyme digested the tissue around the primordial oocytes, leaving them free to be removed. The oocytes were then matured in a second culture medium for a further two weeks. The experiment did result in live young, but the success rate was far from encouraging: 190 eggs cleaved successfully after attempted IVF, but just two of them implanted. Only one of these gave rise to a live baby mouse. What does this mean for infertile women, or those about to become prematurely infertile through treatment for cancer? If this technique is perfected and applied to humans, frozen—thawed ovarian tissue could be a source of large numbers of eggs. As well as helping patients who are about to undergo radiotherapy or chemotherapy, this could also benefit 'typical' IVF patients. A small amount of tissue taken from an ovary, by laparoscopy, could prove to be an altogether more satisfactory source of eggs than the superovulation and needle aspiration used today. It would avoid the need for down-regulating and ovulation-inducing drugs. In the future, it could also produce enough eggs to give patients perhaps a hundred or more embryos from which to choose. Using pre-implantation genetic diagnosis, a couple could be assured of the healthiest embryo possible from the combination of the two partners' DNA.

Dr Adrian Lower thinks that work on maturing eggs outside the body is 'vitally important. I think it's the next major advance in reproductive medicine that we will see over the next five to ten years.'

The technique of maturing eggs from frozen–thawed ovarian tissue would also be another way – in addition to embryo freezing – of offering women the chance to delay having children until late middle age. Unlike patients undergoing cancer treatment, discussed above, such people would not have to worry about the re-introduction of cancerous cells when the graft is performed. Embryologist Jacques Cohen explains the possibilities:

> 'So what you can do is, when you are eighteen years old, take a little piece of ovarian tissue – work done in animals by Roger Gosden and his team – and simply store it so that once you are forty-five, or even fifty-five or sixty – if society changes and the average age becomes ninety or a hundred-and-ten which is going to happen – then if you're ready to become a mother you just have that little piece of ovarian tissue transplanted to your own ovaries.'

Single women in particular may benefit from the technique of ovarian grafts: with embryo freezing, a male partner must be involved. Where embryos are stored long-term, custody battles can ensue if the couples split up. Such cases have already occurred, but could be avoided if eggs could be obtained from frozen–thawed ovarian tissue and fertilized with sperms, frozen or fresh. Women other than cancer patients have had pieces of ovary removed and cryopreserved, for use later in life. Banks of frozen ovarian tissue have already been set up in several centres, including Monash University. These tissue banks have already started collecting ovarian tissue, both for research purposes and in anticipation of medical applications, with pre-treatment cancer patients particularly in mind. Similar options could be offered by the freezing of eggs. While the freezing of sperms and embryos has good success rates, freezing of eggs has proven notoriously difficult throughout the history of cryopreservation; only a small number of births have resulted from eggs that have been frozen. It was generally thought that the size of the human egg – in fact the relatively large volume of water inside it – were to blame. But James Stachecki of the St Barnabas Medical Centre, New Jersey, USA, had a different idea. He thought that the problem might lie with the salt (sodium chloride) solution normally used in cryopreservation. He was aware that the small size of sodium ions present in the solution means that they can pass through the cell membrane, effectively poisoning the egg. So, in 1998, he developed a new approach to freezing eggs. Instead of freezing them in salt solution, Stachecki tried using a solution of a protein called choline. Molecules of choline are too large to pass through the cell membrane into the egg. The results were encouraging: as many as 90 per cent of the eggs survived cryopreservation in Stachecki's solution. The surviving eggs were fertilized, and more than half grew to the blastocyst stage. At the time of writing, these experiments, too, have only been carried out with mouse eggs.

Cellular surgery

Another new technique that may benefit some women is cytoplasmic transfer. The cytoplasm, that surrounds the nucleus of an egg, contains proteins that are vital to the functioning of the cell. In particular, there are many thousands of tiny objects called mitochondria. A mitochondrion is like a power station, providing all the energy the cell needs to stay alive and to develop. A deficiency or imperfection in the proteins or the mitochondria, or in some cases a simple lack of enough cytoplasm, can be a cause of infertility. The idea behind cytoplasmic transfer is to inject healthy cytoplasm from an egg donated by one woman into the egg of a second. A single sperm from the partner of the second woman is injected into the recipient egg at the same time, so this is really a variant of ICSI. The fertilized egg (zygote), now has all it needs to develop normally. In November 1997, a team led by Jacques Cohen, also at the St Barnabas Medical Center, reported the first ever birth of a child after the egg from which it grew received cytoplasm from another woman's egg. Cohen has described the procedure as like 'old-fashioned surgery, just on the cellular level'.

Some newspaper headlines at the time the first pregnancy was announced made much of the idea that the child had two genetic mothers. Indeed, there are pieces of genetic material present in cytoplasm, and some of them would have been transferred from the donor to the recipient egg. Their function is to help make the proteins that are necessary for the healthy functioning of the cell. In fact, this may be the reason that cytoplasm transfer works in the first place; these pieces of genetic material from the donor cytoplasm enable the recipient egg to manufacture the proteins it needs to develop normally after fertilization. During the sixth week of the first pregnancy achieved with the help of cytoplasm transfer, the genetic identity of the foetus was checked, using early amniocentesis in conjunction with DNA fingerprinting. Jacques Cohen explains:

'[The child] had two mothers when it was a zygote and a four-cell embryo. That embryo had two mothers – if you can speak about mothers then – at the eight-cell stage, and maybe when it was a little blastocyst. Maybe even when it was an early foetus. We don't know. But certainly once we tested the cells after amniocentesis, we couldn't find traces of [anything] from the donor.'

In any case, it is the DNA in the nuclei of egg and sperm that determines the genetic identity of the child that developed, and not fragments of genetic material in the cytoplasm. Since that first birth, there have been many more, though not enough to constitute a full clinical trial or to have investigated further why the technique seems to work. Many people who have heard of cytoplasmic transfer assume that it was designed to help older women, whose eggs are defective. This is not the case: defects in older women's eggs are usually found in the chromosomes within the nucleus. Cytoplasmic transfer was simply developed to help women with eggs that do not develop normally after fertilization. The first woman to give birth after cytoplasmic injection was thirty-nine, and had been through four failed attempts at IVF. She is the sort of patient who typically might be able to benefit from the procedure.

What next?
In this chapter, we have looked briefly at some of the recent developments in ART that both push back the frontiers of modern biological and medical science and appeal to new categories of patient. They are helping infertile men and women, or those about to become so, to achieve what they want, as well as bringing more choices to those who are not necessarily infertile. Peter Brinsden, medical director of Bourne Hall IVF clinic, believes in a measured approach to the rapidly developing field of ART. Who knows where it may lead? He says:

'[We should] tread very cautiously I think, and progress very cautiously, as we are with spermatid injection in this country. I think as we will be with cytoplasmic transfer or nuclear transfer or things that might lead on to cloning, I think we need to tread very carefully.'

Chapter 11

CLONING, CLONING, CLONING . . .

'If I'm in a happy marriage, or I'm with a partner that's prepared to stay with me for life, then if the chance came up, I would be the first person to do it because I've always wanted a child and I would do anything to get one, and if it means being the first person ever to have a cloned child and to live with that, then that's what I will do.'

A woman to whom cloning may offer the only chance of a child of her own.

Most assisted reproductive technologies (ARTs) aim to fulfil the desire that many people have to bring up children who are genetically related to them. For some people, cloning may offer a new way of achieving this, and may one day become an accepted technology offered to certain infertile couples. In some cases, it may be the only way that a couple can realize their dream of having their own child. We shall see how this might be true later in this chapter. First, it is necessary to explain what cloning is, and explore some of its potential applications and implications.

Human cloning involves the use of genetic information in a single cell to create a new human being. A baby is normally created by the combination of two 'sex cells', an egg and a sperm. Sex cells, also called germ cells, contain half a set of chromosomes (twenty-three in all). The combination of two germ cells, to form a fertilized egg, makes a new cell with a complete, unique genetic identity (genotype). A fertilized egg contains forty-six chromosomes. Any cell other than a sex cell, called a somatic cell, also contains forty-six chromosomes. So, each somatic cell contains a copy of the complete genotype of the person. The aim of cloning is to use the entire genotype of a single somatic cell to produce a new human being. Therefore, cloning can make a new baby without fertilization. And the baby will have the same genetic identity as the person whose cell was used to make it.

Over the past few decades, the idea of cloning has increasingly become part of public consciousness, and has stimulated the popular imagination. Science fiction books have been written, and films made, on the subject, and these have helped to raise awareness of some of the ethical issues that cloning brings. The ethical questions surrounding cloning are more fundamental than with any other ART. Many people find the concept of human cloning abhorrent, and feel that it should be banned. At the time of writing, no one has gone through with human reproductive cloning, although someone almost certainly will – perhaps they already have as you read this. It is almost certainly that imminent: the technology already exists, as was publicly demonstrated on 23 February 1997. On that day, cloning became international headline news, as 'Dolly' the sheep made her first public appearance.

Dolly was produced from a single cell taken from an adult ewe. John Bracken, one of the team who created Dolly, admits that it was he who thought up the name: 'I said that we should really call her after the well-known country and western singer Dolly Parton, as Dolly herself was derived from mammary cells.'

Dolly was the first ever clone of an adult mammal. So great is her status in the history of reproductive biology that she will be stuffed after her death, and put on display in Edinburgh at the National Museum of Scotland – the country where she was conceived and born. But Dolly was not the first clone of an animal; and certainly not the first ever clone. All plants can be cloned easily, for example – gardeners routinely take cuttings or make grafts. In this sense, cloning is an ancient practice. For some plants – those that reproduce asexually – cloning is perfectly natural, and is in fact the only way for genetic information to pass from generation to generation. A spider plant (Chlorophytum), for example, develops arching stalks, at the end of which grow 'plantlets'. These are small versions of the main plant, which can become free of their stalks to grow as independent copies (clones) of the parent plant. Indeed, the word 'clone' comes from the Greek word *klon*, meaning 'twig'. The plantlets of Chlorophytum are all genetically identical to their 'parent' – their cells carry exactly the same genetic information, or genotype, in their DNA. Many other plants reproduce asexually, too.

Evolution of an asexually reproducing species is slow, since there is no variation in its genotype from generation to generation; but it does happen when random mutations enter the genotype. This lack of variation, from generation to generation, makes asexual reproduction important in horticulture; it ensures a consistent crop. Even species of plant that do not normally reproduce asexually can be made to do so, by grafting parts of a parent plant on to standard 'root stocks', for example. Cloning a particular variety can give the consistent results expected by modern consumers. For example, Thomson seedless grapes all grow on vines that are clones of one plant selected many years ago. Likewise, all individuals of the main variety of banana plant, called Gros Michel, are clones of a selected plant of the same name, which grew in the West Indies in the 1930s. Crossing two plant varieties that have favourable characteristics leads to new strains; the best can be selected and then cloned. The word 'clone' can apply to individual plants that have a genetic double, or to a group of genetically identical ones. In the same way, 'clone' may refer to an individual bacterium, or a whole colony of identical, asexually reproduced bacteria. And in humans, one identical twin is the clone of the other, but a whole set of identical twins, triplets or quads is also referred to as a clone. Identical twins are formed when an embryo breaks into two pieces inside the fallopian tube or the womb. As with the plantlets of a spider plant, identical twins carry the same genotype as each other (although in humans, it is different from their parents' genotypes).

At this point, an idea may come to mind: can a human embryo, produced by IVF, be purposely split apart, to produce human clones? Jerry Hall and Robert Stillman at the George Washington University Medical Center asked the very same question, and set about finding an answer. In 1993, the researchers split apart early embryos, and surrounded each fragment with an artificial zona pellucida. They chose embryos that were not viable and therefore had no chance of implanting. This made the experiment less ethically sensitive than if they had used viable embryos. Some of the embryos developed to the thirty-two-cell stage, before being destroyed. This experiment really was an example of human cloning, but was in truth no more than 'assisted twinning'. A similar experiment was carried out by one of the early pioneers of cloning, Hans Spemann, as long ago as 1902. Spemann used a hair to split a two-celled salamander embryo in half. Two normal, but identical, salamanders were produced by this experiment (developing in a culture dish, as salamanders don't have wombs). Spemann proposed, correctly, that before a certain stage of development, the cells in an embryo are 'undifferentiated'. As explained in Chapter 1, differentiation is the process by which a cell becomes specialized; it is an important part of the development of an organism. A skin cell is 'programmed' to behave differently from a muscle cell, for example. All the cells of an early embryo are undifferentiated, and so do not correspond to any particular tissue in the final animal. This is why Hall and Stillman's experiment, and Spemann's before it, worked. It is also why natural twinning results in two complete organisms, and not two halves. In 1998, a team led by Alan Trounson used a similar technique to turn a single cow embryo into 500 of them. While embryo splitting, by definition, can only involve embryos, nuclear transfer would enable people to produce clones from adult animals.

Dolly the sheep was produced by this nuclear transfer, rather than by embryo splitting; it's a process that has no equivalent in nature. Spemann tried nuclear transfer, too, though he was using embryos. In 1928, he carried out an ingenious experiment designed to prove that the nucleus carries the information that is essential to the development of an embryo. He began by tying a piece of hair tightly around a fertilized salamander egg, effectively making two cells. The nucleus was in just one section of this 'double cell', and could not pass across to the other side. The half with the nucleus developed normally, into a sixteen-cell embryo. At that stage, Spemann loosened the hair, allowing the nucleus to transfer across to the other side of the double cell. He then tied the hair extra tight, to split the single cell into two. The half that now contained the nucleus, which had previously been inactive, went on to develop into a separate embryo. The two embryos were of course genetically identical: they were clones. It was only because Spemann had transferred the nucleus from an undifferentiated cell, which formed part of an early embryo, that development could continue normally into a second embryo. The nucleus of a differentiated cell would have been programmed to behave in a specific way, and would have resulted in, at best, a culture of differentiated cells of one type. But because the nucleus was taken from a cell in an embryo, the second cell acted like a fertilized egg. Most cells of an organism contain the organism's complete genotype.

So how does differentiation work? How are different cells 'programmed' to behave differently from each other, despite having the same genotype? One of the important features of the process is the attachment of proteins to the DNA in a cell, blocking off some genes and enabling others to 'express' themselves. This was the main obstacle to be overcome before the cloning of Dolly could be achieved. One cannot simply inject the nucleus of a differentiated cell into an egg and expect to see the growth of undifferentiated, embryonic cells that would grow to form a lamb.

In 1952 Robert Briggs and Thomas King cloned cells taken from frog embryos. They, too, used nuclear transfer: the nuclei of cells from the frogs' embryos were removed and transferred to unfertilized eggs. In this case, each egg, which received a nucleus, had previously had its own nucleus removed. Such a cell, with its nucleus removed, is said to be 'enucleated'. Some of the eggs grew into normal embryos, and some even into tadpoles. However, when Briggs and King repeated the experiment with nuclei from differentiated cells, they found that the few embryos that developed were deformed. This result led many to believe that it would be impossible to clone an animal from a differentiated cell; that the genetic information was diminished as cells became more specialized. Dolly is proof that this idea is false.

Spawning an index
In 1962 John Gurdon, at Oxford University, UK, carried out experiments similar to those of Briggs and King. The difference was that the nuclei he transferred were taken from the cells of an adult frog. This went against the findings of Briggs and King – that cloning was not possible from fully differentiated cells. And so some scientists challenged Gurdon's results, causing some controversy. For example, some suggested that Gurdon had used undifferentiated cells, which can exist in frogs' intestines. Whether Gurdon succeeded in cloning frogs from adult cells or not, his experiments did attract wide interest, from both within and beyond the confines of the scientific community. So the concept of clones – and in particular, the prospect of human cloning – began to find expression in popular fiction, reaching its height during the 1970s.

The most celebrated, and perhaps most cautionary, tale was *The Boys from Brazil*, written by Ira Levin. It told the story of the multiple cloning of Adolf Hitler by Nazi doctor Josef Mengele. In the story, Mengele produced ninety-four clones of Hitler, and arranged for them to be adopted. When the boys were old enough, they would be taken away from their adopted families, and encouraged to think and act just like the original. It would be Mengele's way of regaining and redoubling power for the Third Reich. Of course, your genotype does not determine your beliefs or the subtleties of your behaviour. These qualities depend to a great extent on your environment, the experiences of your upbringing. And so, the argument goes, if Hitler was cloned, there is no reason why the clones would be anti-Semitic and dictatorial. Levin addressed this argument. In the story, Mengele arranged for certain key events from Hitler's life to be replicated in the boys' lives. For example, the boys' fathers were to be killed at sixty-five, the same age as Hitler's father was when he died. In the end, the plot was foiled by a 'Nazi hunter' who had worked out Mengele's intention. The film version of the tale was released in 1978 – the same year as Louise Brown was born. Also in that year, American author David Rorvik wrote *In His Image: the Cloning of a Man*. The book was put forward as a work of fact – a documentary – and in it Rorvik claimed that a rich executive had paid to have himself cloned, using the technique that Gurdon had employed in 1962. Rorvik was later forced to admit that the story was a hoax. Nonetheless, cloning had certainly been injected into popular culture. Keith Campbell, who was part of the team that created Dolly, recalls his growing interest in cloning:

'I came across the work of John Gurdon, and that fascinated me; that you could take nuclei from later developmental stages, effectively from the cells lining the gut in the tadpole, take that genetic material and put it back into an egg. . . and end up with an adult frog. At about the same time, in about 1984 I saw a lecture at Sussex University by a Swiss scientist called Karl Illmensee, who talked about cloning in the mouse.'

Illmensee had published his work in 1979, and another controversy had ensued. Illmensee reported that he had used nuclear transfer to produce three cloned mice from embryonic cells. We shall probably never know whether Illmensee's claims were true or false – at the time, people were certainly suspicious that he may have fabricated his results. A series of failed experiments had led the scientific community to rule out the possibility of cloning mammals. The public, on the other hand, seemed convinced that it would be possible to clone mammals, including human beings. Irrespective of the truth or falsity of Illmensee's claims, the public were proved right in 1984, when Danish scientist Steen Willadsen took an important, and undisputed, step forwards. Willadsen produced a sheep, by nuclear transfer, from the DNA in an embryonic cell. His procedure was different in two important respects from that used in the previous experiments described earlier. First, he fused an embryonic cell and an enucleated egg cell together, instead of transferring just the nucleus. That technique was pioneered the previous year by Davor Salter and James McGrath at the Wistar Institute in Philadelphia, USA, who had used it with mouse embryos. The second important factor in Willadsen's approach was that he used an unfertilized egg, rather than a fertilized one, as the recipient of the nucleus. This made it easier to carry out the nuclear transfer successfully. But it did mean that the egg had to be 'tricked' into behaving as if it was fertilized before it would develop into an embryo. He placed a single cell from a sheep's embryo next to the unfertilized egg, and fused the two using an electric current. In 1986, while he was working in Texas, Willadsen carried out another experiment, this time resulting in the birth of a calf clone. There was an important difference: the clone was produced from a one-week-old embryo, using a cell that had already partially differentiated. This showed that it really is possible to 'turn back the clock' of a cell, to make it change from a differentiated to an undifferentiated state. The experiment was unpublished, but anecdotal reports of Willadsen's work reached Ian Wilmut, head of the team that eventually produced Dolly:

'The general view was that nuclear transfer would only work with cells from a very early embryo indeed – about eight or sixteen cells. What he had shown was that he could get nuclear transfer to work from an embryo with perhaps 250 cells. He'd broken a barrier.'

The science of the lambs
The cloning procedure that produced Dolly was begun as part of a project that was already ongoing. Wilmut was working at the Roslin Institute in Edinburgh, Scotland. He was looking at ways of introducing specific new genes into the genotype of sheep. These genes, if they became incorporated into the sheep's DNA, would produce useful proteins that are difficult to produce in large quantities in any other way. The sheep were to become living factories producing chemicals such as medicines. (This is an example of genetic engineering, the potential application of which in humans is discussed in Chapter 12.) Wilmut's initial approach did not involve cloning. He would inject specific pieces of DNA – the new genes – into large numbers of embryos, hoping that the genes would be incorporated. This process was successful, but only in some of the embryos. A small number of these would establish pregnancies once transferred to a ewe's womb, and fewer still would go to term and produce the

desired 'transgenic' sheep. So, the procedure was inefficient, and sheep's embryos were not in great supply. When he heard of Willadsen's work, Wilmut hit on a new approach for his own project; cloning could be just what he needed. He would try to insert the new gene into normal cells instead of embryos. If only a small proportion of the cells took up the new gene, it would not matter, as normal cells can be taken from an adult in abundance and so are not in such short supply as embryos. Those cells that did take up the new gene could then be cloned, producing a limitless supply of the altered embryos, and a reliable way of producing transgenic sheep. Wilmut sees an irony in these origins of the cloning project:

'So the reason we started the cloning project was actually to have a way of making genetic changes in animals rather than to be able to make exact copies of animals that we have already.'

Wilmut gained government and private finance, and set about putting together a project team. One of the key members was Keith Campbell, who had studied the 'cell cycle' for his PhD. The cell cycle is the process by which ordinary cells divide, during growth or to replenish tissue. Skin cells are constantly falling off, for example, but they are constantly being replaced, too, by new cells. A new cell does not arise from nowhere: it is produced by an existing cell copying itself and dividing into two, during the cell cycle. One part of the cycle, which proved to be vital in the cloning project, is called G0, or 'gap zero'. At this stage, cells are inactive, or quiescent. Campbell explains:

'The cell cycle is the life cycle of a cell. . . when it duplicates all of its components. So it sort of goes round and round in a circle. It goes through these processes, divides; goes through the processes again, divides. In early embryos, and also during development, cells can sort of exit, leave this cell cycle and go into a resting, or quiescent, phase.'

In 1994, at the University of Wisconsin, Neal First was carrying out a cloning experiment involving cows. He had inadvertently 'starved' the cells he had prepared in a culture dish, and he noticed that they had gone into the quiescent phase. The team at the Roslin Institute decided to starve cells in their culture dishes on purpose, Wilmut remembers:

'The alternative which Keith came forward with was to stop the cells by making them inactive in this particular state. And initially we did it simply for reasons of convenience; so people could sit in the lab, work with exactly the same population of cells without doing anything to them for hours, and know that they were still the same. After we'd been doing that for maybe a month or so, he'd been thinking about this and we had an absolutely critical conversation, when he pointed out to me that these cells might be different, not only in that they were stable, but also they might be different in their response to nuclear transfer.'

The DNA in the nucleus of a cell in the G0 stage can be 'reprogrammed', by the proteins in the cytoplasm of the egg cell, to behave as it would in a fertilized egg. It no longer behaves as DNA in a skin cell, or a muscle cell; or, in the case of Dolly, a cell from a mammary gland. Campbell reasoned that, for the cloning experiment to work, the two cells involved should be 'synchronised': they should both be at the G0 stage. The precursor of the set of experiments that brought Dolly into the world showed that this approach really could work. In 1995, they produced five lambs from part-differentiated cells from sheep's embryos. Unfortunately, three of the lambs died, but the two survivors, called Morag and Megan, were normal, healthy sheep. This was an important achievement, but is often overlooked; everyone remembers the name 'Dolly'.

After their success with Morag and Megan, the team decided to try to obtain clones from other cell types. The began early in 1996, using cells from three different sources: a nine-day-old sheep's embryo, a twenty-six-day-old sheep's foetus, and, most importantly, the mammary gland of a six-year-old ewe. At the time, the team at the Roslin Institute was working collaboratively with a company called PPL Therapeutics, also in Edinburgh. The researchers here were investigating the effect of inserting a gene into cells from a sheep's mammary gland. So this was the source of the mammary cells, although the cells used in the experiment had not been altered. Wilmut and Campbell grew a 'cell line' – by making the cells replicate many times in a culture medium. A total of 277 of the adult mammary cells were successfully fused with enucleated, unfertilized sheep's eggs. The eggs were obtained with the use of gonadotrophin hormones like those used in standard IVF treatment. The resulting 'fused couplets' were incubated in sheep's fallopian tubes in the laboratory, and then any that developed were transferred to the wombs of recipient ewes. After a few weeks, ultrasound scans confirmed the existence of some pregnancies. Keith Campbell remembers the period leading up to the birth of Dolly and the lambs produced from the other cell types:

> 'We used to spend our nights from eleven o'clock till five-thirty in the morning sleeping on the floor down where the sheep were housed and getting up every hour just to go and see if they started to go into labour. Well, you could say it was sod's law – all the lambs were actually born in the day, so we needn't actually have been doing it.'

Dolly was born at 5pm on 5 July 1996. Bill Ritchie, a member of the team at the Roslin Institute, remembers the birth:

> 'In lots of ways it was just a classic birth, in that the lamb was on its feet and trying to suckle and doing the usual things that lambs do: you know, falling over, struggling up and trying again to get on to the teat and eventually you could see that it had connected and its little tail was waggling and that usually means that things are all working well and that the lamb's taking its first suck.'

Only one of the 277 fused couplets involving mammary cells had produced a lamb: not a good success rate. There were seven other lambs, from the other two cell types, but Dolly was by far the most important. She was the first mammal ever to be produced by the cloning of an adult somatic cell (and not by the combination of sperm and egg). The team had to keep quiet about their success for more than seven months, while they prepared their scientific paper – published in the journal *Nature* on 27 February 1997 – and observed the development of the lambs. But when the news broke, a few days before the publication, the silence soon ended. Dolly was an instant global celebrity. Newspapers from around the world sent reporters and photographers, television and radio crews came to visit, and the President of the USA, Bill Clinton, made a broadcast live from grounds of the White House.

Ian Wilmut remembers it: 'Well, he was just one of a number of people, I mean the Pope, a whole range of people sort of sat up and took notice.'

People took notice because this was an incredibly important achievement, with political and medical consequences as well as scientific ones. Later the same year, a genetically engineered sheep clone, Polly, was born at the Roslin Institute. She was much more relevant to the original aims of the plan, and her creation was perhaps more controversial than Dolly's. She was not only the result of cloning: her genotype had actually been altered. However, neither Polly nor Morag and Megan before her attracted as much publicity as Dolly. This sheep became a symbol of the possibility of human cloning. If an adult sheep can be cloned, then there really is nothing in the laws of nature to prevent an adult human being from being cloned. And so all the hypothetical debates over cloning, as well as the science fiction stories, suddenly became very real and very relevant.

Do you copy?
President Clinton immediately called for a moratorium on human cloning, and imposed a ban on federal funding of projects related to it. He asked the US National Bioethics Advisory Commission to prepare a report, with recommendations on how to proceed with this ethically challenging area. The report came out in June 1997, and stated that the Commission had, not surprisingly, 'discovered that the potential ability to clone human beings through the somatic cell nuclear transfer techniques raises a whole host of complex and difficult scientific, religious, legal and ethical issues'.

The Commission advised Clinton to uphold the moratorium on human cloning. And, given the uncertainties about the consequences of cloning, most scientists would certainly impose their own. There are dangers – both known and as yet unforeseen – inherent in the technology of human cloning, at least as it stands today. The procedure that brought about Dolly's existence was very inefficient, for example. A high proportion of the foetuses in the experiment developed abnormally, with weakened organs for example, and were killed in the womb. The thought of doing this routinely with humans is not one to relish. At the rate of progress in the field, however, the safety and efficiency of the technique are likely to be greatly improved. This is why the experiment has ramifications that extend far beyond the particular technique developed at the Roslin Institute. Indeed, in July 1998, scientists working at the University of Hawaii in Honolulu announced that they had produced three generations of mouse clones, reporting a greater success rate. They had used brain cells, and cells from the testes of mice, as the donors of genetic material. These cells are naturally suspended in the G0 state, and this made it easier to synchronize the cells before nuclear transfer, improving the success rate. The Honolulu technique used direct nuclear transfer, rather than fusion of two cells, and this also seemed to increase the success rate. Many other animals have been cloned since Dolly, and the success rate seems to be improving rapidly. In the future, the success of the technique is sure to improve yet more, and the creation of new animals, or humans, by the cloning of adult cells could become routine.

As we have seen, cloning is a natural phenomenon – in twinning and in species that reproduce asexually – so can it be wrong? Why should scientists, politicians, theologians and the general public fear this technology, even if it were applied to human beings? Just what are the religious, legal and ethical issues that human cloning raises?

On a practical, short-term basis, it is important to consider the welfare of the first human clone – he or she would receive a thousand times the publicity of Dolly, for example. There is the issue of identity: a human clone would have no genetic parents in the normal sense, since the egg from which it would grow would never have been fertilized. In a statement issued by the Vatican in 1987, it was claimed that a new human individual's life begins at fertilization. There would be no fertilization in the creation of a human clone. Dolly's genotype was created a generation before she was born, and the same would be true of cloning in humans. Consider an analogy with a spider plant. A clone's single 'parent' – genetically, an identical twin – is the equivalent of a spider plant, while the clone itself is the equivalent of a plantlet that has gained independent existence. And yet no one would claim that different spider plants, or identical twins, are not separate individuals.

Some people fear cloning for the same reason that some people feared IVF – because it is unnatural. These people think that it is wrong to tamper with nature, which is complex and self-regulating, and which we do not yet fully understand. Could we, by tampering with our own evolution, somehow threaten it? On the other hand, does the fact that cloning of adult human beings is unprecedented in nature necessarily make it morally wrong? If human cloning offers advantages to individuals – infertile couples, for example – then perhaps it would be morally wrong not to allow it. In addition to the general objection to cloning on the basis of the fact that it is unnatural, there are many other, more specific objections. In the UK in 1997, the HFEA and the Human Genetics Advisory Commission (HGAC), put out a joint consultation document, 'Cloning issues in reproduction, science and medicine'. In response, the All-Party Parliamentary Pro-Life Alliance put together a comprehensive document, which they published in April 1998. Like other pro-life supporters, they considered cloning unethical because it involved the direct manipulation of human embryos. They expressed many other reasons why they were opposed to human cloning:

> 'We hold that the creation of a human clone would be unethical. In summary, this is because those creating the clone are in an unacceptable position of control over the clone. . . To create a human being as a manufactured creature, with its characteristics decided to suit the ends of others, is an affront to human dignity and a threat to human freedom.'

In their document, the Pro-Life Alliance referred to the scenario explored in Aldous Huxley's novel, *Brave New World*, written as long ago as 1932. Huxley's novel envisages a society in which people are manufactured in cloned 'batches' labelled alpha, beta, gamma and delta. Each category has precisely determined characteristics. The so-called 'alphas' are intelligent, and seek mental stimulation. They become the political leaders, philosophers and so on. The 'deltas' are born with much lower intelligence, and carry out menial tasks, without ever complaining. The society is stable, and everyone is 'happy', and yet its citizens have no real freedom. The pro-life document explores some disturbing possibilities which human cloning could bring about, including one that has parallels with Huxley's vision of dystopia. They imagine a factory owner who uses his money and power to produce multiple clones from a worker with low intelligence and low expectations. He produces a workforce which, like the original cloned worker, is loyal and hard-working. This would be an infringement of human rights, they assert.

But does the possibility of cases like this mean that we should ban cloning outright? It is the factory owner's desire for greater profits that brings about this infringement of rights and freedom, not cloning itself. Like any other technology, cloning is a tool that can be used for good or evil. So, are there ways in which human cloning may be advantageous? We shall explore this question below. Another objection to cloning relates to the treatment of the clone. Pressure might be put on clones to behave in the same way as their 'originator'. A clone of a gifted musician, for example, might disappoint his or her family if he or she showed no interest in music. Clearly in this kind of situation, the 'parents' would have to be counselled as to this possible outcome.

Mother or twin sister?

Whether or not we are heading towards a Brave New World, the routine cloning of human beings would certainly demand a fundamental shift in the public perception of human parent–child relationships. Is the woman who gives birth to her own clone that child's mother or twin sister? And how is that woman's father related to the clone – father or grandfather? Some would argue that we need to review our perception of human relationships in the modern world anyway. The concepts of 'mother', 'father' and 'child' have been the basis of most family relationships as long as there have been families. However, there is nothing to say that it is the only way, or the right way; several variations on this theme already exist, including adoption and surrogate motherhood.

There are many other arguments against reproductive human cloning, in addition to the ones noted above. Even the scientists who created Dolly came out against the use of the technology in human reproduction. Ian Wilmut again:

> 'I think that the emphasis in a lot of the debate, particularly in the United States, is on the rights of the adults to reproduce in the way that they want. I think personally that somebody's got to ask: "Is it in the interests of the child?", and in that particular case I would say it is not and so I personally would disapprove of [human reproductive cloning].'

Perhaps the question of whether cloning is right or wrong simply depends upon what it will be used for. What might be people's motives for being cloned? The most obvious one is perhaps egotistical: cloning offers the ultimate satisfaction of the desire to have children 'in your own image'. In 1998, Iraqi leader Saddam Hussein is reported to have asked his top scientists to clone him. The problem is, of course, that he would have no guarantee that the clones would grow up to be any more like him than a child produced in the normal way. Even if the clones were brought up in exactly the same way as Saddam was, the development of personality and behaviour depends on so many factors. Existing techniques of mind-manipulation will for now be as successful and far more convenient than cloning for those who want to create people who think as they do. Nevertheless, people might still want to use cloning to produce offspring who are related to them. Most heterosexual couples would probably prefer to bear children that are related to both partners. Homosexual couples cannot produce a child that is a genetic combination of both partners (at present anyway). Single people are in a similar position. Might they benefit from cloning? Would it be wrong to produce, say, two children in a homosexual couple, one cloned from each partner? Again, this is not natural, but is it wrong? For couples in which one partner does not produce sex cells, the only option at present is for the fertility clinic to find a donor – of eggs or sperms. The resulting child is related to only one partner. This same result could be achieved using cloning, but without the use of a donor. Again, the couple could have two children, one a clone of each.

There are countless individual scenarios in which cloning could hep to fulfil people's desires to make babies. A woman whose child is killed might want to produce another child identical to the original one – particularly if she has lost the father of the child, too. Again, there might be pressure on the clone to be just like the lost child. A similar case involves women who have ectopic pregnancies, in which the embryo implants in the fallopian tube rather than in the womb. Such pregnancies are normally terminated, either naturally or artificially. Would it be acceptable to take cells from the foetus, and clone them, so that the woman could be given the chance to 'try again' with the same child? This would certainly reduce the disappointment that women feel in such circumstances, and there would have been no first child to emulate.

Is there anyone who would carry out human reproductive cloning simply out of profound curiosity, or to make a name for themselves? There are several people who have stated publicly their intention to produce the first human clone. One of them is American IVF doctor Richard Seed, who pioneered a non-IVF version of embryo transfer during the 1980s. Severino Antinori, the Italian IVF doctor who famously enabled a sixty-two-year-old woman to give birth, has also stated his serious intention to be the first to achieve human cloning. More bizarre is a company called Clonaid, set up by the 'Raelian' religious cult, headed by Claude Vorilhon in Montreal, Canada. Members of the cult believe that cloning carries with it no dangers to humanity, and that aliens used the technology to achieve the resurrection of Jesus Christ nearly 2000 years ago. The company carries out research into cloning, and has offered to clone people for $200,000 each. It has not yet been successful.

If notoriety is the only reason for cloning, then the procedure will almost certainly constitute an infringement of the rights of the clone. Cloning could open the door to another infringement of a right: the right not to reproduce. A single cell taken without permission – while someone is sleeping, for example, could be used to make a clone. Famous athletes or intellectuals might be the targets. Again, it is the intention that is at fault here, not the technology. Banning human cloning would not prevent unscrupulous people from carrying out the technique, so what is the point of banning it? The answer is that a law against cloning illustrates a society's condemnation of it. On the other hand, the absence of such a law is, in effect, a statement of acceptance. In the same way, there are laws against murder but people still commit it. But a law banning human cloning outright might also affect other people: those who could benefit from it without compromising anyone's rights or freedom. At this point, an important distinction must be drawn – between reproductive cloning and therapeutic cloning. For the same techniques that make it possible to create children who are clones could be used manufacture tissues that could be of great benefit to medicine. This will be explored in the final chapter.

There are other potential medical benefits of cloning, some of which promise future developments in assisted reproductive technology. Ian Wilmut describes one of them:

> 'It is suggested that one day it will be possible for a couple who know that they carry a genetic error – perhaps both of them carry the genetic error – to produce an embryo in the usual fun way, or perhaps in the IVF lab, to grow out cells from that embryo, to use precise genetic techniques to correct that error, use cloning to make a new embryo, and then you have a baby which is exactly the same as the original would have been but without that genetic disease.'

And so, while a clone produced from an adult human being may well be some way off, related techniques may help infertile couples or those carrying inherited diseases to obtain a healthy child. The potential benefits are persuading many scientists who were initially set against human cloning to come out in favour, at least of therapeutic cloning. The feeling in the scientific community is beginning to change. There are more concerted efforts to achieve therapeutic cloning, and many scientists who were initially in favour of an outright ban are now suggesting that at least therapeutic cloning should go ahead.

IVF pioneer Robert Edwards thinks that the big questions, about the possible wider implications of cloning, are premature:

'What we need is 10,000 mouse Dollys and 10,000 cattle Dollys, then we'll be nearer the mark to know what's going to happen. By the way these will come, it won't take long to produce the mice; thousands of mice. But I think asking all these questions at the present time is misleading, because you're forced into making decisions on things you don't know, and I think it's wise to keep well within the bounds that you're reasonably certain about.'

Perhaps for now cloning will continue to find uses only with animals. Cloned livestock could give the meat and dairy industries new ways of guaranteeing the quality of their products. But cloning goes beyond farming. In 1997, a research project was set up at the Texas A & M University in the USA. Called the Missiplicity Project, it stems from the desire of a rich executive to clone his dog, Missy. Despite the non-scientific nature of the overall aim, the project has several serious scientific goals, including discovering more about canine reproduction. Another possible application of cloning is saving endangered species. In 1998, the last remaining member of a species of cow was cloned on Enderby Island, New Zealand. The technology could even bring back particular animals that died years ago: providing some cells still remain.

Now that cloning is on its way to being perfected and accepted for use in livestock and pets, is there such a great leap to its routine use in humans? Where would such a leap take us? To Chapter 12.

Chapter 12

BABY-MAKING FUTURES

'I just want to make babies with you.'
Godley and Creme, B-side to 'Wedding Bells'

The technology of baby-making has come a long way since Robert Edwards and Patrick Steptoe developed IVF. SUZI and ICSI (sub-zonal insemination and intracytoplasmic sperm injection) have increased the success rate of IVF, and made it available to more couples, particularly those where the male partner has a low sperm count. PGD (pre-implantation genetic diagnosis) gives new hope to carriers of genetic diseases. The age-old desire to choose the sex of your child has also been addressed, through high-tech sperm selection. The technology of cloning might one day help couples – or individuals – to make a baby of their own.

Despite these advances, the success rate of IVF is still not as high as infertile couples would like – many patients still go without their desired 'take-home baby', even after several attempted treatment cycles. Also, these treatments are still prohibitively expensive for many couples who could benefit from them, apart from where state assistance is available. PGD has not yet found widespread application, partly due to its high cost and partly due to the high levels of skill required by those carrying it out. And human cloning is not likely to find widespread application for some time, and then only if the outcome of important ethical debates allow it to. However, all of these technologies are likely to become more efficient, cheaper and more widespread in the near future. Furthermore, the range of choices for people who want children of their own will continue to grow – there will always be a market for reproductive technology. But does this mean we are heading towards a society where reproduction is simply a matter of consumer choice? In fifty years' time, will people be able to make 'designer babies', manufactured to their specifications?

Whatever the long-term future of reproductive technology, a short-term goal must be to increase the success rate of IVF treatments. Some hope may be offered by a procedure developed at the Colorado Center for Reproductive Medicine in Englewood, Colorado. In 1997, the centre's director of research and development, David Gardner, reported that his team had more than doubled the chance of an embryo implanting in a patient's womb – from 21 per cent to more than 45 per cent. The chance that a pregnancy would result from an embryo that did implant increased from 47 to 63 per cent. What was the secret of this success? Simply to delay transfer of the embryos until they were five-day-old blastocysts. The reason that Gardner decided to try this approach is that embryos do not naturally reach the womb until they are four or five days old. IVF doctors normally transfer embryos after two days; but at this stage in natural reproduction, embryos would still be in the fallopian tubes and would not be ready to implant. Unlike a very early embryo, a blastocyst consists of two distinct types of cell: an inner mass, from which the foetus develops, and an outer layer, which forms the placenta. The placenta attaches the embryo to the lining of the womb. So this would explain why normal IVF – in which embryos are transferred before this outer layer has formed – might suffer from the reduced chance of implantation. To make their approach work, the Colorado team had to take into account the changing needs of an embryo during its first five days. So they kept the embryos in one culture medium for the first forty-eight hours, and then moved them to another for the remaining seventy-two.

Is this the way forward? Some IVF doctors think not. They would prefer to transfer the embryos sooner, not later, than two or three days after fertilization. This would ensure that the embryos were in the most suitable 'culture medium' – the patient's body – as early as possible. The most effective method is sure to be found, and IVF will become more successful, and hopefully cheaper, as a result.

Another short-term or medium-term goal of IVF is to eliminate the need for drugs that stimulate a female patient's body to produce many eggs in the same cycle. Whether or not the use of such drugs increases the risk of ovarian cancer, it does put pressure on a patient's body, as well as playing havoc with her emotions. Also, the drugs make up a large proportion of the cost of IVF, so leaving them out would make IVF more affordable. So some doctors and researchers are investigating ways of carrying out IVF without superovulation. One approach is to stick to 'natural cycle IVF' –

simply not administering the drugs. The problem is, of course, that IVF doctors would then only have one egg per cycle to work with. This would be fine if the success rate per embryo could be increased to 100 per cent. Another approach is to mature eggs from ovarian tissue. This would involve a woman undergoing a laparoscopic procedure to remove small pieces of ovary, which could be frozen until needed. From the biopsied tissue, as many eggs as required – perhaps a hundred or more at a time – could be matured when needed. As an extension of this idea, those that are successfully fertilized could then be subject to pre-implantation genetic diagnosis (PGD), to select the most 'desirable' embryo. The chosen one could even be cloned, so that effectively the same embryo could be transferred every month until a pregnancy resulted. Maturing human eggs outside the body, PGD and cloning human embryos have not become routine yet but, at the rate of progress in the technology of assisted reproduction, all are likely to become so in the foreseeable future. Perhaps this is one way in which cloning may play a part in the future of assisted reproduction.

Mummy, mummy

Cloning could help to satisfy other baby-making desires, too. Chapter 11 mentioned how cloning could help homosexual couples have children of their own. In the case of lesbians, at present each child that a couple has is genetically related to one of the partners – sperm must be donated. It is currently fairly common for a male friend of a lesbian couple to donate sperm for donor insemination, or for the couple to visit a clinic that will carry out the insemination. Cloning offers a way for lesbian couples to have a baby that is not related to a male donor, since sperms are not needed in the cloning process. Even better, both women could be the child's mother, in a very real sense. How?

As cloning involves transferring the nucleus of a 'somatic' cell – a skin cell, for example – into an egg cell, the somatic cell would come from just one partner, who would be the genetic 'parent' of the child. The egg could come from the other woman. If this second woman were to carry the resulting embryo to term, then she would be the biological mother.

This is all very well for lesbians, but what about gay men? At present, the best they can hope for is to agree on a surrogacy arrangement. Again, the resulting child is related to only one of the partners. Cloning would only go as far as eliminating the genetic link to someone outside the couple – the baby would still only be related to one partner. Perhaps some way may be found to form a new genotype (genetic identity) from a combination of both partners' chromosomes. This could also benefit lesbians, of course. This truly artificial method of conception has not seriously been proposed, and, if it is possible at all, is a long way off. If it were to happen, perhaps the best way would be to use the chromosomes from two sex cells (eggs or sperms), which are already halved in number compared with somatic cells. Just as in natural fertilization, a new genotype could then be created by combining the two halves. Attention would have to be given to the sex chromosomes in the case of gay men. The complete genotype of a man includes one X and one Y chromosome. Each sperm, with half the genotype, contains either an X or a Y, so combining two Y-bearing sperms would result in an embryo with two Y chromosomes. If such an embryo could survive to term, it would probably result in a horribly deformed baby, as there are many important genes on the X chromosome. However, in the future, perhaps it will be possible to tell, with absolute certainty, whether a particular sperm is X- or Y-bearing, and therefore to make this process work. Even if this process is theoretically possible, the foetus will still have to be carried by a surrogate. This comes with a risk that the surrogate will not release the baby after carrying it for nine months. In addition, it is more difficult, at present at least, for gay men to arrange a surrogacy than for a married hetero-sexual couple.

Is there a way around this problem? Is it possible for a man to carry a child, for example? Surprisingly, the answer may be 'yes'. Evidence is provided by 'abdominal pregnancy'. Fertilized eggs that escape from the fallopian tubes have been known to implant and establish pregnancies elsewhere in women's abdomens. This is rare and dangerous, but it does happen. As long as the biochemical environment is acceptable, an embryo can implant anywhere inside a body. Homosexual men, as well as transsexuals or the husbands of women who cannot carry children, might benefit from this one day in the far future.

Womb with a view

Another, less physically challenging, possibility is ectogenesis – pregnancy outside the body. The idea of 'bottled babies' is worlds apart from the concept of 'test-tube babies'. And yet some work has already been carried out on developing artificial wombs. The aim of this work is not to provide an outright substitute for the natural womb. Instead, artificial wombs are being designed to be used in the same way as incubators – to keep alive very premature babies. In the early 1990s, a group at the University of Tokyo developed a double-layered rubber womb, filled with artificial amniotic fluid and supplied with nutrients, and kept at a carefully controlled temperature. In 1992, a goat foetus was taken from its mother's womb at 120 days old – equivalent to about twenty-two weeks in a human foetus – and was transferred directly to the artificial womb. It was 'born' out of the rubber womb seventeen days later. If artificial wombs are perfected, then at some point in the future it could be possible to make the whole baby-making process occur outside the body. Eggs would be matured and fertilized *in vitro*, and the resulting embryos transferred to an artificial womb, where they would stay until delivery. The cloned batches of people in Aldous Huxley's *Brave New World* were born from artificial wombs. So is this a technology to fear? If wombs were available commercially, then there would be nothing to stop people who had enough money from producing armies of clones to act as willing slaves or as copies of themselves.

Therapeutic cloning

Not all human cloning would have reproductive aims. Therapeutic cloning, for example, could make human tissue grafts or organ transplants more routine and more successful. One of the main difficulties with transplant operations is rejection – an immune reaction in the recipient's body that treats the foreign tissue as an infection and destroys it. A donor is said to be compatible if the tissue he or she donates is not rejected by the recipient's body. Close relatives are more likely to be compatible than unrelated individuals, and so compatibility is a function of how close individuals are in terms of genetic identity. The ideal donor, then, is generally an identical twin, if one exists. Cloning technology could effectively produce a limitless tissue bank, from which a transplant patient could obtain tissue of any type, with his or her genetic identity, and therefore guaranteed to be compatible. This does not mean the manufacture of a headless copy of a person to act as a donor – an identical twin in the deep freeze. Instead, it means the culturing of human cells that can be made to form any kind of tissue. The medical potential for a culture of such cells would be enormous. In addition to providing a source of tissue for transplant in cases of, say, kidney failure, they could make skin grafts for burns victims, and grafts of nervous tissue for those suffering from Parkinson's disease, Alzheimer's disease or a stroke. One day they could even be the source of complete new organs or limbs.

Two questions come to mind: first: 'Might such cells really exist?' And second: 'What do they have to do with cloning?' The answer to the first question is 'yes', these cells do exist. They are called human embryonic stem cells (hES cells). These cells are normally found in the inner part of a blastocyst. They eventually become a foetus and then a complete human being, so it is clear that these cells really do have the potential to become any type of human tissue. Given the right biochemical signals, hES cells can become skin, muscle, and even brain tissue. And in November 1998, James Thomson at the University of Wisconsin, Madison, USA, announced that he had discovered a way to generate and propagate hES cells. In answer to the second question, human cloning would be an essential part of the process. To make tissues that were compatible with a particular patient, the hES cells used would need to be genetically identical to that patient. So, they would grow from cells taken from the centre of an embryo produced by cloning the patient.

Changing genes

Whether used for reproductive or therapeutic goals, cloning is one genetic technology that is set to shape our future. Some people are rather excited by the possibilities it opens up, while others are fearful of its moral consequences. Another genetic technology that brings both excitement and fear is genetic engineering. We saw in Chapter 11 that shortly after Dolly was born, another cloned sheep, Polly, came into the world. Polly's genotype was not an exact copy of that of her 'mother', however. It had been altered, by the insertion of a human gene that makes a protein that helps to clot blood. So, Polly's milk contained 'human blood clotting factor', but in every other way she was a normal ewe.

Is it possible and worthwhile to use this sort of genetic engineering in human beings? Genes are already inserted into people's bodies in some medical treatments, known as gene therapy. Sufferers of cystic fibrosis, for example, have a defective copy of a gene that is supposed to make an important protein found in the lungs. The wrong gene coding means the wrong protein structure, and the lungs of cystic fibrosis sufferers do not function properly. If a non-defective copy of the gene is inserted into a sufferer's body, it should make the protein and therefore alleviate the disease's symptoms. The genes used in gene therapy are normally injected in a serum or inhaled in an aerosol. In some cases they may be carried by a 'vector' – normally a harmless virus that will help to insert the gene into the DNA of the patient. This approach is known as somatic gene therapy, because the gene is inserted only into somatic cells. It is generally a little 'hit-and-miss': even if copies of the gene do become embedded within some cells, they are not often replicated when cells divide to replenish. However, it is the only genetic manipulation that those already born can hope for – their genotypes have already been determined, at fertilization, and cannot be changed in every cell.

For a long-term eradication of a genetic disease, 'germ-line therapy' might offer a more effective solution. In this treatment, the 'healthy' gene would be inserted into germ cells – eggs and sperms – of sufferers of a disease. The resulting fertilized eggs, embryos, foetuses and people would be free of the genetic disease. Alternatively, the same result could be achieved by a process similar to the one that led to the creation of Polly. The starting point could be cells from an embryo with a genetic disease; the healthy gene would be inserted into these cells. Any embryonic cells that incorporated the new bit of DNA would be cloned, to produce a new human being identical to the adult but without the disease. Germ-line therapy of any form is currently banned, because it would affect the genetics of future generations. However, if it were to eradicate crippling genetic diseases, can it be right to ban it? On the other hand, lifting a ban on germ-line therapy would open the door to non-therapeutic genetic manipulation. For example, could an embryo be genetically altered to be more intelligent, more good-looking or more athletic?

Designer babies are out of reach of present-day technology. To make them a reality, if that is desirable, we would first need to know every detail of human DNA – the entire 'human genome'. DNA is a long, complex molecule, and all along its length are much smaller molecules, called bases. There are four types of base, normally referred to as A, C, G and T (for adenine, cytosine, guanine and thymine). About 3,000 million bases make up the entire human genome. An analogy with computers is useful in explaining how the bases carry information. The '0's and '1's (called 'bits') in a personal computer are arranged in groups of eight, according to a code called ASCII (American Standard Code for Information Interchange). Each group of eight bits is called a byte, and each byte represents a letter, a number or a simple instruction. The letter 'r', for example, is represented inside a personal computer by the byte '01110010'. Individual letters join together to form words. Inside a personal computer, then, a word is represented by a string of bytes. For example, the word 'letters' is represented by the following long string of bits:

01101100011001010111010001110100011001010111001011110011

Amazingly, the bases along the length of DNA are also arranged according to a code, called the genetic code. Bases along the length of DNA do not represent letters or numbers (although some groups of bases do represent instructions!). Instead, they code for chemicals called amino acids, which are the building blocks of proteins, just as letters are the building blocks of words. (The main function of DNA is to carry information on how to build proteins, which in turn make living things.) A sequence of three bases represents a particular amino acid, just as a sequence of eight bits represents a particular letter or number. For example, the sequence 'ACC' represents an amino acid called tryptophan, and 'ATA' represents tyrosine. So, a protein called haemoglobin (see Chapter 7), which consists of more than 140 amino acids, is represented by:

GTGCACCTGACTCCTGAGGAGAAGTCTGCCGTTACTGCCCTGT
GGGGCAAGGTGAACGTGGATGAAGTTGGTGGTGAGGCCCTGG
GCAGGCTGCTGGTGGTCTACCCTTGGACCCAGAGGTTCTTTGA
GTCCTTTGGGGATCTGTCCACTCCTGATGCTGTTATGGGCAACC
CTAAGGTGAAGGCTCATGGCAAGAAAGTGCTCGGTGCCTTTAG
TGATGGCCTGGCTCACCTGGACAACCTCAAGGGCACCTTTGCC
ACACTGAGTGAGCTGCACTGTGACAAGCTGCACGTGGATCCTG
AGAACTTCAGGCTCCTGGGCAACGTGCTGGTCTGTGTGCTGGC
CCATCACTTTGGCAAAGAATTCACCCCACCAGTGCAGGCTGCC
TATCAGAAAGTGGTGGCTGGTGTGGCTAATGCCCTGGCCCACA
AGTATCAC

This very sequence is in *your* DNA – unless you have sickle cell disease. In this latter case, the sequence will appear with just one of the 438 bases interchanged for another. Since 1990, top geneticists have been engaged in a mammoth task – to work out the whole sequence of 3,000 million bases along the human genome. The Human Genome Project was instigated in the USA by the Department of Energy and the National Institutes of Health, but is now being carried out by thousands of scientists in more than twenty countries. It will take a total of about 30,000 person-years to complete, but – with so many working on it, and the increasing use of computers and robots – it should be complete by 2005.

Of course, different people have different genotypes, and so will have differing sequences of bases. But the genotypes of two unrelated individuals are more than 99.9 per cent the same, and all the genes occur in the same positions on each chromosome. The Human Genome Project aims to produce an accurate 'map' of the human chromosomes, and ultimately to find the codes for all the versions of each gene present. Even now, you can look up thousands of genes – as strings of As, Cs, Gs and Ts like the one above – published in databases on the Internet. John Sulston of the Sanger Centre in Cambridge, UK, thinks it is important that the information collected by the Human Genome Project is made available in just this kind of way:

'What we're doing is to collect this vital information – this very powerful, important and valuable information – in the public domain. And what that means is that we're releasing it freely and openly all the time. It's freely available for discussion – no one person, no industry, no government, no individual has special rights over it. In this way I think we can use the information properly.'

The impact of the Human Genome Project on the future of medicine and reproductive technology is likely to be profound. It will enable new drug and gene therapies to be tailor-made to specific diseases or even specific patients. The ethical, legal and social implications of the project are huge. When combined with DNA chips, which can look for specific sequences of bases in fragments of DNA, the information collected by the Human Genome Project opens up the question of genetic screening (raised in Chapter 7). Insurance companies would be very interested in this sort of information, and there might be portable DNA readers in every doctor's surgery. Genes have been discovered whose incidence is correlated with many and varied human conditions. In 1993, Dean Hamer at the National Institutes of Health, USA, claimed to have found the 'gay gene' for example. Most genes that code for complex traits, rather than simple physical characteristics, work in concert rather than singly, and so such traits cannot simply be 'eradicated'. Furthermore, these polygenetic traits also depend largely on the environment. There are genes that have been discovered (and located on the human chromosomes) that are connected with colon cancer, cystic fibrosis, breast cancer and many more.

The Human Genome Project will probably not bring designer babies in your lifetime. But further in the future, when genetic engineers really can confidently tinker with sequences of human DNA, in germ-line manipulation, the possibilities are mind-blowing. Then we might have the power to make babies with a good chance of being geniuses or athletes. Of course, if and when genetic engineering is more routine and costs less, it is still likely that it will only be the rich who will be able to afford it. The richest parents will be able to afford to have the 'best' designer babies, which will have the very best opportunities – both in their genes and in their education and home environment – to be successful. And so, in turn, they will become rich (while others become relatively poorer, both financially and genetically?). Most importantly, this trend will be cumulative, so that children in any particular generation will have the benefit of any 'positive' changes that their ancestors have made to their family's genetics. They can also choose to make their own changes that will benefit their own children – and their children's children. The divide between rich and poor is likely to open up wider than ever.

Whether this scenario really develops, no one will know, but it has already been convincingly portrayed in the film *Gattaca* (notice the title is formed from only the letters A, C, G and T). In the nearer future, the gap between rich and poor – in terms of what they can hope for in and for their children – looks likely to continue to widen anyway. And this will certainly be true of reproductive choice. How many people in the poorest countries of the world have tried even one IVF cycle? But as long as people have the means to spend thousands of pounds buying, say a car, there will certainly be a market for reproductive technologies.

As for the question of designer babies, perhaps a basic and long-standing human desire will render it unnecessary, and will limit the extent of genetic manipulation to curing disease. Most loving couples' overwhelming desire is to have children who are the result of a combination of their own genes. That has always been the driving force behind making babies.

GLOSSARY

allele a specific version of a gene. All genes have more than one allele.

amniocentesis a form of prenatal genetic testing, in which some of the amniotic fluid that surrounds a developing foetus is taken for analysis. The technique can diagnose some genetic or chromosomal abnormalities, including Down syndrome.

biopsy the surgical removal of living tissue. This includes the removal of one or two cells from a human embryo, during pre-implantation genetic diagnosis (PGD).

blastocyst a fairly well-developed embryo, consisting of two distinct layers. The inner layer goes on to become the foetus, while the outer layer becomes the placenta.

chromosome one of the DNA-containing objects in the nucleus of a cell. The somatic cells of a human being each contain forty-six chromosomes: twenty-two pairs and two sex chromosomes.

cryopreservation the freezing of embryos, eggs, sperm or other reproductive tissue, for later use.

culture a substance or mixture of nutrients in which living tissues can grow in a laboratory. An embryo can be kept alive for a number of days 'in culture'.

cytoplasm the substance contained within a cell, surrounding the nucleus, but not including it. Cytoplasm contains nutrients and 'organelles' essential to the functioning of the cell.

differentiation the process by which the cells of an embryo develop into specific tissues, such as skin cells, muscle cells and brain cells.

DNA deoxyribonucleic acid. It is a chemical substance that carries information from generation to generation. Chromosomes are made of DNA.

down-regulation a medical treatment that stops a woman's normal monthly cycle. It is one of the initial stages of conventional IVF treatment.

embryo the stage of development from conception until foetus.

foetus a developing baby. An embryo becomes a foetus after the end of the second month of pregnancy.

FSH follicle stimulating hormone. This causes an oocyte to mature in a Graafian follicle in women and stimulates sperm production in men.

gamete a sex, or germ cell (an egg or a sperm).

gene a specific length of a chromosome, consisting of DNA. The DNA of a gene holds the instructions for making a specific protein. Your body is largely made of proteins.

genotype the complete DNA of a particular living thing. Each individual human being has a very similar, but unique, genotype.

germ cell the same as gamete.

Graafian follicle a fluid-filled cavity in an ovary, in which an oocyte matures. The follicle develops around the oocyte, and deteriorates if no pregnancy is established.

hCG human chorionic gonadotrophin, a hormone produced by the placenta. A test for hCG is therefore the basis of the standard pregnancy test.

hormone chemicals that control the body. They are released by various organs, and they play important roles in reproduction.

ICSI intracytoplasmic sperm injection. In this process, an attempt is made to fertilize an egg by directly injecting it with a single sperm.

implantation the attachment of an embryo to the lining of a woman's womb. It usually signifies that a pregnancy is established.

laparoscope an instrument that can be used to investigate or carry out abdominal surgery. It is inserted through a small incision in the abdomen.

nucleus the central part of a cell, which contains the chromosomes.

oocyte an immature egg. A woman is born with a lifetime's supply of oocytes. Normally one oocyte is released from one of her ovaries every month, at ovulation.

oogenesis the process by which an oocyte matures, to become an egg.

PCR polymerase chain reaction. This is a cunning biochemical reaction, the result of which is multiple copies of DNA. This means that PGD can be carried out accurately on even the DNA from a single cell.

PGD pre-implantation genetic diagnosis. The process involves the biopsy of typically one cell from an embryo. Analysis of the DNA contained within the cell can determine whether or not the embryo is likely to develop a genetic disease.

placenta the tissue that connects the developing foetus to the lining of its mother's womb.

polar body a small cell produced when an oocyte matures, during the process of oogenesis. The polar body contains half a set of chromosomes, but very little cytoplasm.

sex chromosome a chromosome of either type 'X' or 'Y'. Somatic cells of a female each have two X chromosomes, while those of a male have an X and a Y.

somatic cell any cell other than a gamete.

spermatid an immature sperm.

superovulation any technique that increases the number of eggs released by a woman's ovaries, from the normal one per month, to as many as thirty.

SUZI sub-zonal insemination. In this process, an attempt is made to fertilize an egg by injecting several sperms into the space between the egg cell's membrane and the zona pellucida.

zona pellucida (zona) the outer coating that surrounds an egg. Sperms pass through the zona before they reach the egg's cell membrane, which they must penetrate to achieve fertilization.

zygote a fertilized egg.

INDEX